T0324685

Pharmaconutrition and Nutrition Therapy in Critical Illness

Guest Editor

PAUL E. WISCHMEYER, MD

CRITICAL CARE CLINICS

www.criticalcare.theclinics.com

Consulting Editor

RICHARD W. CARLSON, MD, PhD

July 2010 • Volume 26 • Number 3

SAUNDERS an imprint of ELSEVIER, Inc.

W.B. SAUNDERS COMPANY
A Division of Elsevier Inc.

Elsevier Inc. • 1600 John F. Kennedy Blvd., • Suite 1800 • Philadelphia, Pennsylvania 19103-2899

http://www.theclinics.com

CRITICAL CARE CLINICS Volume 26, Number 3
July 2010 ISSN 0749-0704, ISBN-13: 978-1-4377-2436-3

Editor: Patrick Manley
Developmental Editor: Donald Mumford

Critical Care Clinics (ISSN: 0749-0704) is published quarterly by Elsevier Inc., 360 Park Avenue South, New York, NY 10010-1710. Months of issue are January, April, July, and October. Business and Editorial Offices: 1600 John F. Kennedy Blvd., Suite 1800, Philadelphia, PA 19103-2899. Customer Service Office: 6277 Sea Harbor Drive, Orlando, FL 32887-4800. Periodicals postage paid at New York, NY and additional mailing offices. Subscription prices are $167.00 per year for US individuals, $395.00 per year for US institution, $83.00 per year for US students and residents, $206.00 per year for Canadian individuals, $490.00 per year for Canadian institutions, $240.00 per year for international individuals, $490.00 per year for international institutions and $121.00 per year for Canadian and foreign students/residents. To receive student/resident rate, orders must be accompanied by name of affiliated institution, date of term, and the *signature* of program/residency coordinator on institution letterhead. Orders will be billed at individual rate until proof of status is received. Foreign air speed delivery is included in all *Clinics* subscription prices. All prices are subject to change without notice. POSTMASTER: Send address changes to *Critical Care Clinics*, Elsevier Periodicals Customer Service, 11830 Westline Industrial Drive, St. Louis, MO 63146. **Customer Service: 1-800-654-2452 (US). From outside of the US, call 1-314-447-8871. Fax: 1-314-447-8029. E-mail: journalscustomerservice-usa@elsevier.com (for print support) or journalsonlinesupport-usa@elsevier.com (for online support).**

Reprints. For copies of 100 or more of articles in this publication, please contact the Commercial Reprints Department, Elsevier Inc., 360 Park Avenue South, New York, NY 10010-1710. Tel.: 212-633-3813; Fax: 212-462-1935; E-mail: reprints@elsevier.com.

Critical Care Clinics is also published in Spanish by Editorial Inter-Medica, Junin 917, 1er A, 1113, Buenos Aires, Argentina.

Critical Care Clinics is covered in *MEDLINE/PubMed (Index Medicus)*, *EMBASE/Excerpta Medica*, *Current Concepts/Clinical Medicine*, *ISI/BIOMED*, and *Chemical Abstracts*.

Printed and bound in the United States of America
Transferred to Digital Print 2011

Contributors

CONSULTING EDITOR

RICHARD W. CARLSON, MD, PhD
Chairman Emeritus, Department of Medicine, Maricopa Medical Center and Director
of Medical Intensive Care Unit; Professor, University of Arizona College of Medicine; and
Professor, Department of Medicine, Mayo Graduate School of Medicine, Phoenix, Arizona

GUEST EDITOR

PAUL E. WISCHMEYER, MD
Associate-Chairman for Clinical and Translational Research, Director of Nutrition Therapy
Services, Director of Medical Student Research, Professor of Anesthesiology, University
of Colorado at Denver School of Medicine, Aurora, Colorado

AUTHORS

CRAIG M. COOPERSMITH, MD, FACS, FCCM
Professor, Department of Surgery, Emory University School of Medicine, Atlanta, Georgia

CLIFFORD S. DEUTSCHMAN, MS, MD, FCCM
Professor of Anesthesiology and Critical Care; Director, The Stavropoulos Sepsis
Research Program, University of Pennsylvania School of Medicine, Philadelphia,
Pennsylvania

JESSICA A. DOMINGUEZ, PhD
Assistant Professor of Anesthesiology, Department of Anesthesiology, University
of Colorado Denver School of Medicine, Aurora, Colorado

GABRIEL HERRERA, MD
PUH-UPMC, Pittsburgh, Pennsylvania

DAREN K. HEYLAND, MD
Professor of Medicine, Department of Medicine, Queen's University and Clinical
Evaluation Research Unit, Kingston General Hospital, Kingston, Ontario, Canada

RYAN T. HURT, MD
Assistant Professor of Medicine, Division of General Internal Medicine, Mayo Clinic,
Rochester, Minnesota; Departments of Medicine and Physiology and Biophysics,
University of Louisville School of Medicine, Louisville, Kentucky

RICHARD J. LEVY, MD
Division of Anesthesiology and Pain Medicine, Children's National Medical Center,
Washington, DC; Associate Professor of Anesthesiology and Pediatrics, The George
Washington University School of Medicine, The Stavropoulos Sepsis Research Program,
University of Pennsylvania School of Medicine, Philadelphia, Pennsylvania

OLLE LJUNGQVIST, MD, PhD
Professor, Department of Surgery, Örebro University Hospital, Örebro, Sweden

DILEEP N. LOBO, DM, FRCS
Associate Professor and Reader, Division of Gastrointestinal Surgery, Nottingham Digestive Diseases Centre NIHR Biomedical Research Unit, Nottingham University Hospitals, Queen's Medical Centre, Nottingham, United Kingdom

JULIE M. MARTIN, MS, RD, CD
Division of Pulmonary and Critical Care, Department of Medicine, University of Vermont College of Medicine, Burlington, Vermont

KONSTANTIN MAYER, MD
University of Giessen Lung Center (UGLC), Medical Clinic II, Justus-Liebig-University, Giessen, Germany

STEPHEN A. MCCLAVE, MD
Division of Gastroenterology, Hepatology and Nutrition, Department of Medicine, University of Louisville School of Medicine, Louisville, Kentucky

NICOLAS MONGARDON, MD, MSc
Research Fellow, Bloomsbury Institute of Intensive Care Medicine, Wolfson Institute for Biomedical Research, University College London, London, United Kingdom

JUAN B. OCHOA, MD, FACS
PUH-UPMC, Pittsburgh, Pennsylvania

CLAUDE PICHARD, MD, PhD
Nutrition Unit, Geneva University Hospital, Geneva, Switzerland

ALBERT J. RUGGIERI, BS
Department of Anesthesiology and Critical Care, The Stavropoulos Sepsis Research Program, University of Pennsylvania School of Medicine, Philadelphia, Pennsylvania

MERVYN SINGER, MD, FRCP
Professor, Department of Medicine, Bloomsbury Institute of Intensive Care Medicine, Wolfson Institute for Biomedical Research, University College London, London, United Kingdom

RENEE D. STAPLETON, MD, MSc
Assistant Professor of Medicine, Division of Pulmonary and Critical Care, Department of Medicine, University of Vermont College of Medicine, Burlington, Vermont

RONAN THIBAULT, MD, PhD
Nutrition Unit, Geneva University Hospital, Geneva, Switzerland

KRISHNA K. VARADHAN, MSc, MRCS
Research Fellow, Division of Gastrointestinal Surgery, Nottingham Digestive Diseases Centre NIHR Biomedical Research Unit, Nottingham University Hospitals, Queen's Medical Centre, Nottingham, United Kingdom

LINDSAY-RAE B. WEITZEL, PhD
Instructor, Department of Anesthesiology, Translational Pharmaconutrition Research Laboratories, University of Colorado Denver, Aurora, Colorado

PAUL E. WISCHMEYER, MD
Associate-Chairman for Clinical and Translational Research, Director of Nutrition Therapy Services, Director of Medical Student Research, Professor of Anesthesiology, University of Colorado at Denver School of Medicine, Aurora, Colorado

XINMEI ZHU, MD, PhD
PUH-UPMC, Pittsburgh, Pennsylvania

Contents

At present, we are in a "revival" period in clinical nutrition in critical care, especially in the area of "pharmaconutrition." Adequate nutrition may hinge not only on how many calories are provided but also on the ability to provide key pharmacologically acting nutrients. Traditionally, nutrition has been viewed as vital for metabolism, growth, and repair. But, it is now known that some nutrients, when given in therapeutic doses, appear to serve as pharmacologic agents to improve clinically relevant outcomes. Thus, larger therapeutic doses of specific nutrients may be required to replace acute deficiencies brought on by specific injury or disease states. Recent data also imply that the number of calories and protein delivered early in the intensive care unit (ICU) stay has a significant effect on outcome in at-risk patients. It is thought that the future of ICU nutrition will involve administering early nutrition preferentially via the enteral route. Supplementation by parenteral route may be used in at-risk patients when adequate enteral calories cannot be provided. Specific pharmaconutrients can also be administered as separate components, much like a drug is given. Large multicenter trials are planned or are underway to test these hypotheses. The use of basic clinical pharmacology, molecular biology, and clinical research principles in the study of nutritional therapy will lead to answers on how to administer the right nutrients, in the right amounts, at the right time to critically ill patients.

Maintenance of nutritional status is particularly challenging during critical illness. There is a common perception of a race against the clock to adequately feed the patient to prevent or minimize the sometimes catastrophic muscle wasting and general catabolic state that can result in the patient's deterioration. However, the course of critical illness may be separated into 3 phases, each with highly differing metabolic needs. The initial phase, in which the body attempts to fight the acute insult, is generally hypermetabolic. When the body fails to overcome the insult, it enters into a second phase, which is akin to hibernation. This stage is characterized by a functional metabolic shutdown triggered either by a lack of adequate energy supply or perhaps by the direct switching off of metabolism to spare excess use of a dwindling substrate and energy resource. Those strong enough to survive this phase enter into a period of recovery during which appetite returns, anabolism recommences, and organ function is restored. Nutrition should perhaps closely follow these nonlinear requirements, so as to avoid deleterious under- or overnutrition during the appropriate phase. This approach fits a teleologic argument that enabled many sick people to survive well before the advent of modern medicine and explains why catabolism still occurs despite adequate feeding.

The volume of clinical guidelines produced by national and international societies has virtually exploded in the literature over the past decade. The most important aspect of guidelines is transparency, that is, the connection between the recommendation or guideline statement and the underlying supportive studies from the literature should be transparent. Clinical guidelines should help organize the literature, identify key areas of patient management, and provide a framework with which the clinician may operate. The reader of a guideline should embrace controversy, trace back and review the underlying literature, and then determine whether practice should be altered as a result of the guideline recommendations. The purpose of this article is to understand the derivation of clinical guidelines, to learn how to resolve controversy or differences between guidelines and clinical practice, and to learn steps to apply the guidelines to an individual institution or clinical practice.

Total parenteral nutrition was developed in the 1960s and has since been implemented commonly in the intensive care unit (ICU). Studies published in the 1980s and early 1990s indicate that the use of total parenteral nutrition is associated with increased mortality and infectious morbidity. These detrimental effects were related to hyperglycemia and overnutrition at a period when parenteral nutrition was not administered according to the all-in-one principle. Because of its beneficial effects on the gastrointestinal tract, enteral nutrition alone replaced parenteral nutrition as the gold standard of nutritional care in the ICU in the 1980s. However, enteral nutrition alone is frequently associated with insufficient coverage of the energy requirements, and subsequent protein–energy deficit is correlated with a worse clinical outcome. Recent evidence suggests that all-in-one parenteral nutrition has no significant effect on mortality and infectious morbidity in patients in the ICU if a glycemic control is obtained and hyperalimentation avoided. Thus, the time has come to reconsider the use of parenteral nutrition in the ICU. Supplemental parenteral nutrition could prevent onset of nutritional deficiencies when enteral nutrition is insufficient in meeting energy requirements. Clinical studies are warranted to show that the combination of parenteral and enteral nutrition could improve the clinical outcome of patients in the ICU.

The practice of measuring gastric residual volumes (GRVs) has become a routine part of enteral feeding protocols in the critical care setting. However, little scientific evidence indicates that their use improves patient outcomes. The use of GRVs is more of a tradition, which unfortunately guides the delivery of enteral nutrition (EN). The practice of GRVs is predicated on several flawed assumptions. Using GRVs in hospitalized patients assumes that the practice is well standardized, that GRVs reliably and accurately measure gastric contents, and that they sufficiently distinguish normal from abnormal emptying. The practice also assumes that GRVs are easy to interpret, that a tight correlation exists between GRVs and aspiration, and that continuing EN after a high value for GRV is obtained leads to pneumonia and adverse patient outcomes. And finally, clinicians assume that GRVs are an inexpensive "poor man's test" for determining tolerance of EN. This article reviews studies showing the fallacies of these assumptions. Although clinicians are unlikely to stop using GRVs, interpretation of these must be modified so as not to interrupt the delivery of EN. Using a protocol that directs appropriate responses to elevated GRVs should promote the delivery of EN and improve patient outcome.

T cell dysfunction significantly increases susceptibility to infections and organ failure after trauma or surgery (physical injury). This coincides with a persistent drop in arginine availability, a necessary amino acid for normal T cell function. Recent data led to the identification of a novel mechanism of T cell suppression caused by the depletion of arginine through the induction of arginase 1 (ARG1) in a specialized group of immature myeloid cells, now named myeloid-derived suppressor cells (MDSC). In addition to T cell dysfunction, arginine depletion leads to the decrease in nitric oxide (NO) production. Dietary therapy containing arginine at supraphysiologic concentrations along with other components such as omega-3 fat acids, antioxidants, nucleotides, and vitamin A is associated with improvement in T cell function, NO production, and a significant decrease in infection rates. The authors propose that a pathologic decrease in arginine availability is an identifiable nutrition deficiency syndrome that worsens outcomes if left untreated.

Fish oil is rich in omega-3 fatty acids, which have been shown to be beneficial in multiple disease states that involve an inflammatory process. It is now hypothesized that omega-3 fatty acids may decrease the inflammatory response and be beneficial in critical illness. After a review of the mechanisms of omega-3 fatty acids in inflammation, research using enteral nutrition formulas and parenteral nutrition lipid emulsions fortified with fish oil were examined. The results of this research to date are inconclusive for both enteral and parenteral omega-3 fatty acid administration. More research is required before definitive recommendations can be made on fish oil supplementation in critical illness.

Glutamine (GLN) has been shown to be a key pharmaconutrient in the body's response to stress and injury. It exerts its protective effects via multiple mechanisms, including direct protection of cells and tissue from injury, attenuation inflammation, and preservation of metabolic function. Data support GLN as an ideal pharmacologic intervention to prevent or treat multiple organ dysfunction syndrome after sepsis or other injuries in the intensive care unit population. A large and growing body of clinical data shows that in well-defined critically ill patient groups GLN can be a life-saving intervention.

Enhanced recovery after surgery (ERAS) is a multimodal perioperative care pathway designed to attenuate the stress response during the patients' journey through a surgical procedure to facilitate the maintenance of pre-operative bodily compositions and organ function and in doing so achieve early recovery. The key factors that keep patients in hospital after uncomplicated major abdominal surgery include the need for parenteral analgesia, intravenous fluids secondary to persistent gut dysfunction, and bed rest caused by lack of mobility. The elements of the ERAS pathways are aimed to address these issues and the interventions that facilitate early recovery cover all three phases of the perioperative period during the patients' journey. They also provide clear guidance to all members of the clinical team.

The intestine plays a central role in the pathophysiology of critical illness and is frequently called the "motor" of the systemic inflammatory response. Perturbations to the intestinal barrier can lead to distant organ damage and multiple organ failure. Therefore, identifying ways to preserve intestinal integrity may be of paramount importance. Growth factors and other peptides have emerged as potential tools for modulation of intestinal inflammation and repair due to their roles in cellular proliferation, differentiation, migration, and survival. This review examines the involvement of growth factors and other peptides in intestinal epithelial repair during critical illness and their potential use as therapeutic targets.

Sepsis is among the most common causes of death in patients in intensive care units in North America and Europe. In the United States, it accounts for upwards of 250,000 deaths each year. Investigations into the pathobiology of sepsis have most recently focused on common cellular and subcellular processes. One possibility would be a defect in the production of energy, which translates to an abnormality in the production of adenosine triphosphate and therefore in the function of mitochondria. This article presents a clear role for mitochondrial dysfunction in the pathogenesis and pathophysiology of sepsis. What is less clear is the teleology underlying this response. Prolonged mitochondrial dysfunction and impaired biogenesis clearly are detrimental. However, early inhibition of mitochondrial function may be adaptive.

THE CLINICS ARE NOW AVAILABLE ONLINE!

Access your subscription at:
www.theclinics.com

Preface

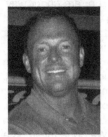

Paul E. Wischmeyer, MD
Guest Editor

"Our food should be our medicine and our medicine should be our food."
—*Hippocrates*

The past 50 years of medicine and critical care have brought great advances in the treatment of disease with novel pharmacologic agents. Largely ignored has been the vital role of basic nutrients and calories in the treatment of critical illness and injury. The shortcomings of our field in delivering nutrition to our sick patients are highlighted by recent data from a worldwide survey of critical care nutrition practice involving nearly 3000 patients. These data reveal ICUs worldwide deliver approximately *50% of the calories we as physicians prescribe* to our patients for the *first 2 weeks of ICU care*.[1] Imagine if you as an ICU physician prescribed 1 g of vancomycin be given daily to your patient dying of MRSA sepsis and you discovered 2 weeks later that only 500 mg were delivered each day? This would never be tolerated, yet this is a daily occurrence in every ICU in the world (except ironically in Burn Intensive Care Units, where perhaps the most severely injured patients in the hospital reside). This travesty of poor critical care nutrition delivery has resulted from years of poorly designed or nongeneralizable trials in the fundamental feeding and nutrition support of our patients. Further, there has been a lack of laboratory-based exploration into the mechanistic science underlying the risks and benefits of nutrition and nutrient administration following injury and illness.

Presently, we are in a "revival" period in clinical nutrition in critical care. This is particularly true in the area of "pharmaconutrition." We have recently discovered that adequate nutrition may hinge not only on how many calories we provide, but also on our ability to provide key pharmacologically acting nutrients. For example, rapid mobilization of amino acids stored in muscle is a vital mechanism for survival following acute illness. These amino acids are used as obligate nutrient sources for the immune system and gut. Recent data indicate that these amino acids also serve as a key stress signals that initiate activation of fundamental cell protective pathways following an insult. For various teleologic reasons, the body becomes rapidly depleted of these substrates and their supplementation may be fundamental for optimal recovery. These data have helped spawn the new field of "nutritional pharmacology."

Crit Care Clin 26 (2010) xiii–xiv
doi:10.1016/j.ccc.2010.05.001
0749-0704/10/$ – see front matter © 2010 Elsevier Inc. All rights reserved.

criticalcare.theclinics.com

The "revival" in critical care nutrition is highlighted by a significant number of new randomized, controlled (often multicenter) clinical trials examining the benefits of nutrition therapy and pharmaconutrition, which have been completed or are under way. These will finally begin to answer the ultimate questions regarding the outcome benefit of various forms of nutrition therapy. Further, mechanistic laboratory advances in our understanding of the role of nutrients as pharmacologic agents are now being translated into focused trials of specific nutrients. These trials examine nutrition's effect on clinically relevant end points, such as length of stay, infectious morbidity, and survival. It is exciting that we have begun to apply basic clinical pharmacology, molecular biology, and clinical research principles to our study of nutrition in critical illness. Thus, the critical care field can look with anticipation to forthcoming answers on how to best use nutrition therapy to improve patient outcomes. We hope these data will finally answer the questions about how to administer the right nutrients, in the right amounts, at the right time.

In this issue of *Critical Care Clinics,* the clinical and mechanistic evidence for optimal delivery of calories and specific pharmaconutrients is reviewed. Key topics reviewed in this issue include how many calories should be fed and by what route, data for the use of specific nutrients, and finally how to evaluate the plethora of often conflicting nutritional guidelines that exist in critical care. Discussions of the evolutionary role of nutrition in critical illness are undertaken and fundamental challenges to long-held paradigms in nutrition (like the use of gastric residuals) are brought forth.

I would like to thank the authors for generously contributing their time and expertise in the preparation of this issue. I would also like to acknowledge the Elsevier editorial staff for their tireless support and patience in bringing this issue to completion. I sincerely hope that this issue serves as a timely and current reference to "reintroduce" critical care practitioners to the importance of nutrition in critical illness and to the rapidly growing field of nutritional pharmacology.

Paul E. Wischmeyer, MD
Department of Anesthesiology
University of Colorado at Denver School of Medicine
12700 East 19th Avenue, Box 8602, RC2 P15-7120
Aurora, CO 80045, USA

E-mail address:
Paul.Wischmeyer@ucdenver.edu

REFERENCE

1. Cahill NE, Dhaliwal R, Day AG, et al. Nutrition therapy in the critical care setting: what is "best achievable" practice? An international multicenter observational study. Crit Care Med 2010;38(2):395–401.

The Future of Critical Care Nutrition Therapy

Paul E. Wischmeyer, MD[a],*, Daren K. Heyland, MD[b]

KEYWORDS

• Pharmacology • Pharmaconutrition • Glutamine
• Arginine • Surgery • Intensive care
• Parenteral nutrition • Enteral nutrition

> *Our food should be our medicine and our medicine should be our food.*
> —Hippocrates

The last 50 years of medicine and critical care have brought great advances in the treatment of disease with novel pharmacologic agents. The vital role of basic nutrients and calories in the treatment of critical illness and injury has been largely ignored. The shortcomings in delivering nutrition to sick patients is highlighted by recent data from a worldwide survey of critical care nutrition practice involving nearly 3000 patients. These data reveal that intensive care units (ICUs) worldwide deliver approximately 50% of the calories that physicians prescribe to patients for the first 2 weeks of ICU care.[1] Imagine if you as an ICU physician prescribed 1 g of vancomycin to be given daily to your patient dying of MRSA sepsis and discovered 2 weeks later that only 500 mg was delivered each day? This situation would never be tolerated; yet this is a daily occurrence in every ICU in the world (except ironically in burn intensive care units, where perhaps the most severely injured patients in the hospital reside). This travesty of poor critical care nutrition delivery has resulted from years of poorly designed or nongeneralizable trials in the fundamental feeding and nutrition support of patients. Further, there has been a lack of laboratory-based exploration into the mechanistic science underlying the risks and benefits of nutrition and nutrient administration following injury and illness.

This work was supported by National Institutes of Health Grants NIDDK- U01 DK069322, NIGMS- RO1 GM078312 to Paul E. Wischmeyer.
a Department of Anesthesiology, University of Colorado at Denver School of Medicine, 12700 East 19th Avenue, Box 8602, RC2 P15-7120, Aurora, CO 80045, USA
b Department of Medicine, Queen's University and Clinical Evaluation Research Unit, Kingston General Hospital, Kingston, ON K7L 2V7, Canada
* Corresponding author.
E-mail address: Paul.Wischmeyer@ucdenver.edu

Crit Care Clin 26 (2010) 433–441
doi:10.1016/j.ccc.2010.04.011   criticalcare.theclinics.com
0749-0704/10/$ – see front matter © 2010 Elsevier Inc. All rights reserved.

THE EVOLUTION OF NUTRITION THERAPY: FROM CAVEMEN TO CRITICAL CARE UNITS

Traditionally, the lack of focus on nutrition as vital therapy in the critical care setting has been because of the observation that in nature acute illness reduces food intake by inducing anorexia, loss of appetite, or simply not permitting the organism to forage for food. At its discovery, tumor necrosis factor α was known as cachexin. This and other cytokines released in the first few hours following stress and injury induces anorexia and catabolism. The early systemic inflammatory response syndrome (SIRS) pathway has been preserved through many years of evolution. Thus, the body uses anorexia and catabolism in the face of stress and injury as a key survival mechanism. However, it must be realized that until the last 150 years, if the proverbial "saber-tooth" tiger attacked you, you had perhaps 48 hours to recover before dying. Even if you survived the initial injury, you were often left behind by your tribe as a liability, for you could not gather food or reproduce and they likely had to carry you, which was less than ideal when other tigers were lurking. Survival from acute injury involved achieving hemostasis and preventing rapid, overwhelming infection. Thus, eating and anabolism were not part of this primal fight for survival. The understanding and management of this survival mechanism has changed dramatically since the evolution of emergency medicine, surgery, and critical care. Now, severely ill and injured individuals are supported through massive insults. Thus, although lean body mass catabolism is mandatory, long-term survival mandates that lean body loss be minimized by early calorie/substrate delivery in the acute phase. Aggressive feeding, and perhaps proanabolic therapy, should follow in the recovery or convalescent phase. Adequate acute care nutrition hinges not only on how many calories are provided but also on the ability to provide key pharmacologically acting nutrients that the body rapidly becomes deficient in after an insult. For example, mobilization of amino acids stored in muscle is a vital mechanism for survival. These amino acids are used as obligate nutrient sources for the immune system and gut. Recent data indicate that these amino acids also serve as stress signals that initiate activation of fundamental cell protective pathways after an insult. This has spawned a new field of nutritional pharmacology.

WHAT ABOUT "AFTER THE ICU"?

In addition to the probable key role of nutrition in survival in the ICU setting following an acute illness or injury, significant mortality occurs after critically ill patients are discharged from the hospital. More than 50% of the 6-month mortality after severe sepsis occurs after the patient has been discharged from the ICU.[2] Recent data reveal that one-third of patients discharged after community-acquired pneumonia are deceased at 1 year.[3] These deaths are believed to occur indirectly as a result of catabolism, loss of lean body mass, lack of therapeutic physical activity, and ultimately weakness and inability to walk.[3,4] These patients often go to rehabilitation centers or go home only to die of pulmonary embolus or pneumonia because they are unable to stand, get out of bed, or perform activities of daily life. Acute care physicians see these patients as a "success" because they survived their acute illness and left the ICU. But, many of these patients ultimately die or have severely limited qualities of life. Thus, ICU physicians must not only provide care for the acute phase of illness with vasopressors, resuscitation, ventilation, and antibiotics to enhance survival but also minimize the mandatory catabolism that occurs during the acute phase and manage the convalescent phase of severe illness, when the key intervention becomes nutrition, anabolism, and rehabilitation.

EARLY AND ADEQUATE CALORIE DELIVERY: WHO SHOULD RECEIVE IT AND ARE WE FAILING?

As many as 50% to 70% of hospitalized patients may be malnourished.[5,6] A recent study emphasizes the importance of providing adequate enteral or oral nutrition to all hospitalized patients.[7] This trial examined hospitalized patients for the occurrence of gut failure or inadequate gut function. Patients with gut failure were defined in this study as those who failed to achieve 80% of goal enteral feeds for at least 48 hours anytime during their hospital stay. Patients diagnosed with gut failure had a mortality of greater then 80%, whereas those able to be fed near goal for at least 48 hours had less than 20% mortality. Gut failure led to significant increases in mortality and sepsis. By univariate analysis, gut failure was associated with a 16-fold increased risk of death.[7]

The key to providing successful nutritional therapy appears to begin with initiation of enteral or oral feeding within 24 to 48 hours of admission to the ICU and appropriate resuscitation. A recent observational cohort study of nutritional practices in 167 ICUs across 21 countries was conducted to evaluate worldwide nutrition practices in 2772 patients.[1] Despite multiple international guidelines recommending early initiation of enteral nutrition in the ICU, we are only successful in delivering approximately 50% of prescribed daily calories for the entire first 2 weeks of ICU admission. In addition, in some major developed countries, such as the United States, it takes more than 60 hours to initiate any enteral feeding at all.

Further, it appears that not all ICU patients are created equal when it comes to the need for caloric delivery. This same multinational observational cohort study used body mass index (BMI, kg/m^2) as a surrogate marker of nutritional status before ICU admission.[8] Regression models were developed to explore the relationship between nutrition received and 60-day mortality and ventilator free days (VFDs), and examine how BMI modifies this relationship. Overall, study patients received a mean of 1034 kcal/d and 47 g of protein per day. There was a significant inverse linear relationship between the odds of mortality and total daily calories received. An increase of 1000 cal/d was associated with an overall reduction in mortality (odds ratio for 60-day mortality, 0.76; 95% confidence interval [CI] 0.61–0.95, P = .014) and an increase in VFDs (3.5 VFDs; 95% CI, 1.2–5.9, P = .003). This beneficial treatment effect of increased calories on mortality was observed in patients with a BMI of less than 25 and greater than 35 with no benefit for patients with a BMI of 25 to less than 35. Mortality was also reduced for every additional 30 g of protein per day given to these patients. This mortality benefit held true after adjusting for acuity of illness and other patient factors. Thus, some patients may benefit a great deal from provision of additional calories early in their ICU stay, while others may not benefit at all.[8] This is key when considering the use of early parenteral nutrition (PN) as a primary calorie source or more appropriately as a supplement to often inadequate enteral feeding. It might be inferred from these data that early use of PN might be of benefit in patients with a BMI of less than 25 or greater than 35. Patients with a BMI of 25 to 35 may not benefit from early PN use; in fact, they may only be exposed to the inherent risks of infection and medical error that PN carries. Several large randomized controlled trials (RCTs) are now planned or are underway to study this question.

NIL PER OS AFTER SURGERY: DOES THIS MAKE ANY SENSE AND DOES IT HURT PATIENTS?

One of the causes of poor early enteral feeding in the ICU and throughout the hospital is the archaic practice of nil per os after surgery. The practices of maintaining prolonged nil per os periods after surgery and awaiting "bowel sounds" to initiate feeding are not supported by clinical or scientific data. In fact, there is now extensive clinical data indicating that the practice of keeping patients nil per os until the return of bowel sounds or passage of gas should be abandoned because it likely worsens clinical outcome including survival.[9,10] This is particularly true in high-risk surgical patients with malnutrition at time of surgery. The fear of anastomotic dehiscence if patients were fed too early has not been confirmed. Clinical trial data reveal that enteral feedings started immediately postoperatively improve anastomotic healing and reduce anastomotic dehiscence.[9,10] The Cochrane review group recently addressed this question by examining the effect of very early enteral feeding versus delayed enteral feeding after gastrointestinal surgery. Their meta-analysis of multiple RCTs revealed that early enteral nutrition led to a 59% relative risk (RR) reduction (RR, 0.41 [95% CI, 0.18–0.93], $P<.03$) of complications after gastrointestinal surgery.[9] Modern thinking preaches that "ileus begets ileus," and the longer one waits to feed after surgery or other injury the greater the chance of persistent gastroparesis and ileus. Burn care provides the most useful example of this phenomenon. Patients in major burn centers with the most massive injury known to be survivable by a human (up to and beyond 90% burns) are fed within hours of admission and tolerate this well. If feeding is delayed even for short periods of time, significant ileus and gastroparesis set in, making feeding more difficult. Thus, if one wishes to consistently be successful in enterally feeding sick patients, early feeding (even if it is only trophic in nature) gives the greatest chance for success. Sufficient early nutritional support of surgical patients not expected to eat soon after surgery has also reduced hospital length of stay (LOS) and decreased costs.[11]

PHARMACONUTRITION: WHAT IS IT AND WHAT IS THE FUTURE?

Nutrition is defined as that physiologic process that involves the assimilation of food necessary for adequate metabolism, growth, and repair. In addition to these traditional functions, some nutrients, when given in therapeutic doses, appear to serve as pharmacologic agents.[12–14] These pharmaconutrients can positively or negatively effect clinical outcome just as any other pharmacologic agent would.[12–14] These larger therapeutic doses of specific nutrients may be required to replace acute deficiencies brought on by specific injury or disease states. In recent years, various single and combination pharmaconutrient therapies have been tested in multiple clinical settings.[12–14]

Complete mechanistic and clinical data for the key pharmaconutrients are discussed in the articles by Weitzel and Wischmeyer, Zhu and colleagues, and Stapleton and colleagues elsewhere in this issue. This article summarizes the key findings that have led to the evolution of pharmaconutrition as a concept. There is now a rapidly growing body of literature that is elucidating each individual nutrient's basic mechanistic effects in the setting of acute illness.[12–16] Three of the well-studied pharmaconutrients are glutamine, arginine, and omega-3 fatty acids. Mechanistically, glutamine is vital to many essential immune functions.[16] Glutamine has been found to induce the heat shock proteins, which are essential to the cell's ability to survive injury and to attenuate the SIRS response during critical illness.[16] Arginine is vital to preventing T-lymphocyte dysfunction following physical injury.[17] Omega-3 fatty acids (specifically eicosapentaenoic acid and docosahexaenoic acid) serve as precursors for resolvins and protectins, which assist in resolution of inflammation and decrease tissue injury.[15] These data indicate that specific nutrients appear to have specific roles following particular injury and illness states. For example, arginine deficiency occurs rapidly after physical injury[17,18] (trauma and surgical injury) but not after sepsis.[17]

The clinical outcome data in more than 30 trials and 3000 patients studied support a significant treatment effect of arginine supplementation to reduce rate of infection (RR, 0.58 [95% CI, 0.48, 0.69, $P<.00001$]) and overall LOS (weighted mean difference, -2.09 [95% CI, -3.20, -0.97, $P = .0002$]) after major surgery versus standard enteral nutrition.[19] However, very little benefit, and perhaps harm, is observed in septic patients.[20] Conversely, glutamine is likely of the greatest benefit in acutely ill patients with sepsis and organ failure, who typically have the most severe glutamine deficiency. Further, this glutamine deficiency at ICU admission has been correlated with increased mortality.[21] Recent data indicate that glutamine therapy is strongly recommended to reduce mortality in patients receiving PN in the ICU, which is supported by a grade A recommendation by all available clinical nutrition guidelines worldwide. These data are taken from 4 level I and 13 level II RCTs totaling nearly 900 patients studied. These studies reveal that glutamine supplemented PN was associated with a significant reduction in overall mortality (RR, 0.71; 95% CI, 0.55, 0.92, $P = .008$). Significant reductions in infection and hospital LOS with glutamine therapy were also observed. The meta-analysis of all RCTs that used glutamine (enteral and parenteral) shows a statistically significant reduction in mortality in ICU patients of all types (21 studies, >1500 patients studied). Thus, glutamine is clearly required for all ICU patients receiving PN and appears beneficial when given enterally or parenterally in other acute care settings (please see www.criticalcarenutrition.com for details).

These data demonstrate that the nutrients being administered must be carefully targeted to the specific type of critical illness being treated (trauma vs infectious sepsis vs postsurgery) (**Fig. 1**, **Table 1**). The stage of inflammatory response of patient must also be considered when selecting specific pharmaconutrients to be given. The immunomodulating mechanisms of the specific nutrients are summarized in **Fig. 2**. Clinical trials of specific nutrients using markers of immune function (such as an arginase I or interleukin 6 level) as entry criteria must be designed. These markers may prove vital to the determination of which patients should be treated using a nutrient with immunostimulating effects (ie, arginine) or antiinflammatory effects (ie, omega-3 fatty acids).

THE FUTURE OF NUTRITIONAL THERAPY IN CRITICAL ILLNESS: A VISION

At present, we are in a "revival" period of interest in nutritional therapy in critical illness, particularly in the area of pharmaconutrition[13] (or nutritional pharmacology). Further, years of poorly designed or nongeneralizable trials in fundamental feeding and nutrition support are being reexplored using modern clinical trial methods and newly discovered mechanistic science.

The vision for the future of critical care nutrition is one where there will be initiation of early (<48 hours post-ICU admit) delivery of nutrition, preferentially via the enteral route, which will be supplemented by PN in at-risk patients when adequate enteral calories cannot be provided. Pharmaconutrients will be administered to target therapy to specific disease states as separate components, much like an antibiotic or drug is given. A validated nutritional assessment tool of biomarkers and other measures will guide this targeting of pharmaconutrients, calories, and nutrition type. The response to pharmaconutrients and calories delivery will also be able to be monitored over time by a validated assessment biomarker. This concept is summarized in **Fig. 3**. In addition, it has to be determined how to evaluate gut function in the sick patient, with biomarkers to assess if the gut is able to function to absorb nutrients. Therapies such as the use of epidermal growth factor (as described in the article by Dominguez and Coopersmith elsewhere in this issue) to protect the gut in patients at risk for gut failure should also be learned.

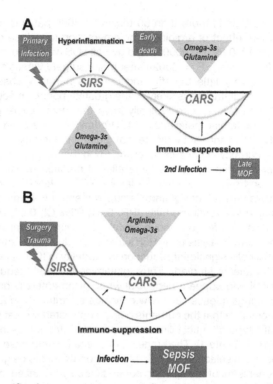

Fig. 1. Role of specific pharmaconutrients on inflammatory response in (A) sepsis/infection and (B) surgery/trauma. SIRS, systemic inflammatory response syndrome; CARS, compensatory antiinflammatory response syndrome; MOF, multiorgan failure.

In the critical care patient, the best resource for evaluating the data for nutrition can be found at www.criticacarenutrition.com. This Web site is a continuously updated repository for all data in the critical care nutrition setting. On a yearly basis all new RCTs in critical care nutrition are added to a rigorous meta-analysis of each key topic. These data form the basis for the Canadian Critical Care Nutrition Guidelines published on this Web site. With the advent of the multidisciplinary critical care team, the best opportunity to provide optimal nutritional care in the ICU is the presence of

Table 1
Clinical effects of immunomodulating nutrients in specific states of critical illness and injury[a]

Nutrient	Infections	LOS	Mortality
Glutamine[22]	↓ Critical illness ↓ Surgery	↓ Critical illness ↓ Surgery	↓ Critical illness
Arginine[18,19] (all studies used arginine as part of "cocktail" formula)	↓ Surgery ↓ Trauma	↓ Surgery ↓ Trauma	↑ (?) Sepsis following infection
Omega-3 Fatty Acids[15]		↓ ARDS	↓ ARDS (?)

Abbreviations: ARDS, acute respiratory distress syndrome; ↓, reduced in.
  [a] Key references listed in the table. Please see www.criticalcarenutrition.com for additional data in critical illness.

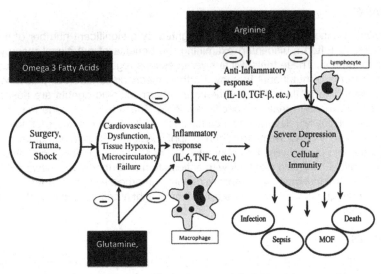

Fig. 2. Mechanism of action for specific immunomodulating nutrients on immune system dysfunction after trauma and surgical injury. IL, interleukin; MOF, multiorgan failure; TGF, transforming growth factor; TNF, tumor necrosis factor. (*Data from* Angele MK, Chaudry IH. Surgical trauma and immunosuppression: pathophysiology and potential immunomodulatory approaches. Langenbecks Arch Surg 2005;390(4):333–41.)

a nutritional therapy team. This team should be made up of dieticians, nurses, and pharmacists who can provide the needed level of assessment, monitoring, and data-driven care to optimize delivery of nutrition to the diverse population of sick patients. It is ideal if a physician trained in nutritional care can direct this team, but this is becoming more difficult to achieve. The paucity of trained nutritional therapy physicians is reaching a crisis level throughout North America.

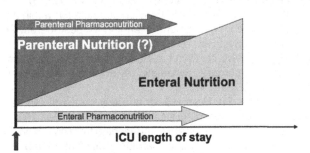

- Assessment of nutritional risk
- Measurement of biomarker(s) to determine which pharmaconutrient/aggressiveness of caloric intake
- Set of tools/biomarkers to monitor response to nutrition/nutrient therapy

Fig. 3. Nutritional therapy for critically ill patients of future.

SUMMARY

The revival in critical care nutrition is highlighted by a significant number of new or ongoing RCTs (often multicenter) examining the benefits of nutritional therapy and pharmaconutrition. These trials will answer questions regarding the outcome benefit of various forms of nutritional therapy. Further, mechanistic laboratory advances in the understanding of the role of nutrients as pharmacologic agents are now being translated into focused trials of specific nutrients. These trials examine the effect of nutrition on clinically relevant end points, such as LOS, infectious morbidity, and survival. It is exciting that we have begun to apply basic clinical pharmacology, molecular biology, and clinical research principles to our study of nutrition in critical illness. Thus, the critical care field can look with anticipation to forthcoming answers on how to best use nutritional therapy to improve patient outcomes. It is hoped that these data will answer the questions on how to administer the right nutrients, in the right amounts, at the right time.

REFERENCES

1. Cahill NE, Dhaliwal R, Day AG, et al. Nutrition therapy in the critical care setting: what is "best achievable" practice? An international multicenter observational study. Crit Care Med 2010;38(2):395–401.
2. Weycker D, Akhras KS, Edelsberg J, et al. Long-term mortality and medical care charges in patients with severe sepsis. Crit Care Med 2003;31(9):2316–23.
3. Kaplan V, Clermont G, Griffin MF, et al. Pneumonia: still the old man's friend? Arch Intern Med 2003;163(3):317–23.
4. Herridge MS, Cheung AM, Tansey CM, et al. One-year outcomes in survivors of the acute respiratory distress syndrome. N Engl J Med 2003;348(8):683–93.
5. Singh H, Watt K, Veitch R, et al. Malnutrition is prevalent in hospitalized medical patients: are house staff identifying the malnourished patient? Nutrition 2006; 22(4):350–4.
6. Baccaro F, Moreno JB, Borlenghi C, et al. Subjective global assessment in the clinical setting. JPEN J Parenter Enteral Nutr 2007;31(5):406–9.
7. Gatt M, MacFie J, McNaughton L, et al. Gut function is an independent indicator of patient outcome: proof of principle. Clin Nutr Suppl 2007;2(2):108.
8. Alberda C, Gramlich L, Jones N, et al. The relationship between nutritional intake and clinical outcomes in critically ill patients: results of an international multicenter observational study. Intensive Care Med 2009;35(10):1728–37.
9. Andersen HK, Lewis SJ, Thomas S. Early enteral nutrition within 24h of colorectal surgery versus later commencement of feeding for postoperative complications. Cochrane Database Syst Rev 2006;4:CD004080.
10. Lewis SJ, Egger M, Sylvester PA, et al. Early enteral feeding versus "nil by mouth" after gastrointestinal surgery: systematic review and meta-analysis of controlled trials. BMJ 2001;323(7316):773–6.
11. Neumayer LA, Smout RJ, Horn HG, et al. Early and sufficient feeding reduces length of stay and charges in surgical patients. J Surg Res 2001;95(1):73–7.
12. Dupertuis YM, Meguid MM, Pichard C. Advancing from immunonutrition to a pharmaconutrition: a gigantic challenge. Curr Opin Clin Nutr Metab Care 2009;12(4): 398–403.
13. Jones NE, Heyland DK. Pharmaconutrition: a new emerging paradigm. Curr Opin Gastroenterol 2008;24(2):215–22.
14. Ochoa JB. Separating pharmaconutrition from classic nutrition goals: a necessary step. Crit Care Med 2008;36(1):347–8.

15. Pontes-Arruda A, Demichele S, Seth A, et al. The use of an inflammation-modulating diet in patients with acute lung injury or acute respiratory distress syndrome: a meta-analysis of outcome data. JPEN J Parenter Enteral Nutr 2008;32(6):596–605.
16. Wischmeyer PE. Glutamine: mode of action in critical illness. Crit Care Med 2007; 35(Suppl 9):S541–4.
17. Popovic PJ, Zeh HJ 3rd, Ochoa JB. Arginine and immunity. J Nutr 2007;137(6 Suppl 2):1681S–6S.
18. Waitzberg DL, Saito H, Plank LD, et al. Postsurgical infections are reduced with specialized nutrition support. World J Surg 2006;30(8):1592–604.
19. Weitzel L, Dhaliwal R, Drover J, et al. Should perioperative immune-modulating nutrition therapy be the standard of care? A systematic review. Crit Care Med 2009;13:132.
20. Heyland DK, Novak F, Drover JW, et al. Should immunonutrition become routine in critically ill patients? A systematic review of the evidence. JAMA 2001;286(8): 944–53.
21. Oudemans-van Straaten HM, Bosman RJ, Treskes M, et al. Plasma glutamine depletion and patient outcome in acute ICU admissions. Intensive Care Med 2001;27(1):84–90.
22. Angele MK, Chaudry IH. Surgical trauma and immunosuppression: pathophysiology and potential immunomodulatory approaches. Langenbecks Arch Surg 2005;390(4):333–41.

The Evolutionary Role of Nutrition and Metabolic Support in Critical Illness

Nicolas Mongardon, MD, MSc[a], Mervyn Singer, MD, FRCP[b],*

KEYWORDS

• Nutrition • Metabolism • Critical illness • Critical care
• Hibernation • Multiorgan failure

Improvements in critical care management enable us to care for patients for prolonged periods that are well beyond their unsupported physiologic capability. It is not uncommon for critically ill patients to require weeks, if not many months, of intensive care. Yet this is a highly artificial, nonphysiologic existence that has only been inflicted on human beings for the last few decades. Humans have not evolved to suddenly cope with extrinsic organ supports, with a decreased conscious level through exogenous sedation, and with abnormal modes of nutrition, be it intravenous or continuous drip feed.

Nutrition is likely to play a crucial role in survival from prolonged critical illness because an adequate substrate supply is at the crossroads of every physiologic system within the body. However, huge uncertainties still persist as to the optimal manner to feed patients. Many aspects of nutritional management are yet to attain a global consensus, as perfectly illustrated by some striking discrepancies between the US[1,2] and European[3] guidelines. Considerations on optimal food intake and composition are discussed in articles by other investigators in this issue. The authors, however, focus on a description of the metabolic modifications occurring during acute

Funding: Dr Nicolas Mongardon is funded by a grant from the "Fondation pour la Recherche Médicale" (FRM). Professor Mervyn Singer receives funding support from the Medical Research Council and the Wellcome Trust. This work was undertaken at UCLH/UCL, which receives a proportion of its funding from the UK Department of Health's NIHR Biomedical Research Centre's funding scheme.
The authors have no potential conflicts of interest related to this article.
[a] Bloomsbury Institute of Intensive Care Medicine, Wolfson Institute for Biomedical Research, University College London, Cruciform Building, Gower Street, London WC1E 6BT, UK
[b] Department of Medicine, Bloomsbury Institute of Intensive Care Medicine, Wolfson Institute for Biomedical Research, University College London, Cruciform Building, Gower Street, London WC1E 6BT, UK
* Corresponding author.
E-mail address: m.singer@ucl.ac.uk

Crit Care Clin 26 (2010) 443–450
doi:10.1016/j.ccc.2010.04.001
0749-0704/10/$ – see front matter © 2010 Elsevier Inc. All rights reserved.

and long-term critical illnesses, with particular emphasis on the implications for nutritional support.

VARIATIONS IN ENERGY EXPENDITURE DURING CRITICAL ILLNESS

In a normal adult, energy expenditure (EE), and thus nutritional requirement, is divided into 3 main components.[4] The first component is basal metabolic rate, which accounts for approximately two-thirds of EE.[5] This energy is dedicated mainly toward maintaining membrane integrity and molecule synthesis, whereas a minor part is consumed by basal organ function. The second component is physical work, representing a quarter of the total EE. Thermogenesis accounts for the third and relatively minor component, accounting for less than 10% of EE, although this proportion may vary markedly between different organs.

EE is highly challenged during critical illness. In addition to the 3 key components described previously, patients also have to cope with alterations in metabolism induced by the injury, whatever its nature, and by the treatments given in response.[4]

The initial insult is, in itself, a major determinant of further EE. Whereas minor elective surgery has relatively little effect,[6–8] major surgery has significant effects with a reported 20% to 40% increase in EE. Trauma results in similar increases, ranging from 20% to 60%.[9–11] As described later, the very early response to an infectious insult is a large increase in metabolism. However, with established sepsis there is a strong negative correlation between energy use and disease severity. Sepsis without organ failure had the highest increase in EE over predicted values (60%), whereas septic shock was associated with EE values comparable to values seen in healthy individuals.[12] Zauner and colleagues[13] also found that on admission to the intensive care unit (ICU), EE was inversely related to severity.

Of note, acute inflammatory conditions such as sepsis or trauma are usually associated with increases in body temperature that also affect EE. For every 1°C rise in core temperature, EE increases by 7% to 10%.[4] Other factors related directly to the initial insult or to subsequent complications may further increase EE, including alcohol withdrawal, seizures, or agitated delirium. Furthermore, many of the unnatural supports administered to patients in ICU also modulate their EE. These supports may range from control of temperature using antipyretics through to therapeutic hypothermia, or rewarming after major surgery. Administration of nutrition itself, either enteral or parenteral, increases EE,[14] as do catecholamine infusions.[4] On the other hand, β-blockers, neuromuscular blocking agents, sedatives, and mechanical ventilation may markedly decrease EE.[15]

Role of Premorbid Conditions

Underlying conditions and comorbidities may also influence EE. For example, obese people have, in general, a higher basal EE compared with thin people; however, they behave in a roughly similar fashion during critical illness. Yet there are marked differences in terms of protein mobilization and fat use.[16] Even though older patients often present with a decreased fat-free, lean body mass and thus a decreased EE than younger people, they still manifest similar endocrine and metabolic changes after elective bowel surgery.[17]

EVOLUTION OVER TIME

Nutritional requirements are made still more complex over time by both changes in endogenous metabolism and altered therapeutic modifications. Changes in metabolism may be typically described by 3 distinct phases (**Fig. 1**).

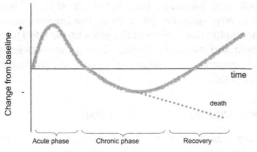

Fig. 1. Proposed schema for the 3 phases of metabolism in critical illness.

The Acute Phase

In this phase, the organism directs its resources toward defending itself against the acute event. Cardiac output and regional blood flow to vital organs, such as heart and liver, are increased, whereas nonvital regions (at least for dealing with acute insults), such as gut and skin, receive less perfusion. A predominantly proinflammatory phenotype is expressed, with hypothalamo-hypophyseal stimulation resulting in marked changes in hormone synthesis and release.[18] The released hormones are predominantly catabolic, such as catecholamines and cortisol. There is also a marked increase in substrate use, although, after available glucose is depleted, glycogen stores are mobilized, lipolysis is increased, and amino acids and lactate are liberated from skeletal muscle for use by other organs. An intense proteolysis may occur, with sarcopenia reaching up to 10% of the total muscle mass within the first week of critical illness.[19] To fuel this stress response and to generate more energy for increased metabolic demands, global oxygen consumption is also increased. Soop and colleagues[20] observed parallel elevations of cardiac output, oxygen delivery, and oxygen consumption within a few hours of injection of lipopolysaccharide into healthy adults.

The Established Phase

The second phase can be described as almost the virtual obverse of the initial acute phase. Here, the hyperdynamic cardiovascular circulation declines an antiinflammatory phenotype predominates, and a state of immunoparesis occurs.[21] Hormonal levels tend to decrease and receptor levels are downregulated. Organ failure becomes established with variable shutdown of different body systems including kidney, gut, and muscle. Notably, these failed organs look, to all intents and purposes, structurally normal with often minimal, if any, evidence of histologic damage.[22,23] Indeed, in a postmortem study of 20 patients who died due to multiorgan failure, Hotchkiss and colleagues[24] found an increase in apoptosis of lymphocytes, gut epithelium, and splenocytes but remarkably little cell death elsewhere. During this period, EE and oxygen consumption are reduced in line with severity, as described earlier. The patient may thus be considered to enter a state akin to hibernation or estivation during this phase of established organ failure, the implications of which are discussed later.

The Recovery Phase

Should the patient survive their critical illness, then their body has to restore an adequate degree of biochemical and physiologic activity in the failed organs that which would be compatible with unsupported function. In addition, the patient has to regain organ bulk and replenish their substrate stores. This last phase thus mandates a heavy energy requirement, with all the body systems endeavoring to return to their premorbid function. EE must therefore be elevated to meet the demands of increased synthetic and muscular activity. During the recovery phase in patients with septic shock, Kreymann and colleagues[12] observed an increase in EE to 161% of predicted requirements.

WHAT DO THESE MODIFICATIONS OF EE REPRESENT?

The core question surrounding all these modifications in EE during the course of critical illness is whether they are pathologic or adaptive. Nature has the striking ability to cope with unfavorable conditions, for example hibernation in situations of severe cold, estivation during excessive heat or drought, and adaptation to hypoxemia during deep-sea diving in some species of turtle. In the medical field, hibernation after myocardial infarction provides compelling evidence of a similar adaptation in humans, with transient dysfunction followed by ad integrum restoration. Histologic appearances comparable to hibernation have also been reported in hearts studied in a septic murine model.[25] The lack of consistent histopathologic changes in failed organs suggests that this hibernation phenomenon may be widespread; the organ may sacrifice its function transiently in the hope of later recovery. Acute renal failure, to which the moniker "acute tubular necrosis" is usually applied erroneously, is another striking example of physiologic shutdown in the face of structural normality to which a severe functional failure cannot be easily squared. Furthermore, failed organs in sepsis generally show a dramatic recovery potential, provided they were not previously damaged through chronic illness or as a consequence of iatrogenic complication. To illustrate this point, none of a cohort of 425 patients who required renal replacement therapy for acute kidney injury became dependent on dialysis.[26] It is also worth noting that organ failure may develop despite adequate perfusion and oxygenation.[27] The decrease in oxygen consumption with increasing severity of sepsis[12] combined with the presence of adequate tissue oxygen tension in resuscitated sepsis[28] implies availability of oxygen at the cellular level but decreased use. As mitochondria are predominantly responsible for the bulk of oxygen consumption, this decrease in oxygen consumption does suggest that mitochondria play a central role in the pathophysiology of organ failure.

To reconcile these elements the authors proposed a theory, in which organ failure represents a functional adaptation rather than a structural pathology.[29] Multiorgan failure could perhaps be perceived as a means by which the body stops expending fuel on expensive and futile functions (at least in the short to medium term) when it is under attack, while maintaining basal metabolism for cell integrity and the minimal biochemical processes necessary for survival. Even if this process leads to complete physiologic failure of the organ, it may preserve the ability for subsequent recovery. This metabolic shutdown is likely to be triggered by mitochondrial dysfunction, although definitive proof is lacking.[30]

If this hypothesis is applied to metabolism and EE in the 3 phases of sepsis described earlier, it can be inferred that the initial hypermetabolic phase is consistent with an attempt to fight and overwhelm the initial insult. However, an insult likely prevails if is too powerful and prolonged. The body thus recognizes that a continued battle may be fruitless and so, in an attempt to survive, it changes strategy by entering a state akin to hibernation. This metabolic shutdown decreases nutrient requirements, reduces substrate use, and lowers EE. This strategy aims to conserve cell survival by sacrificing its short-term functionality. From a teleologic point of view, this would be an entirely appropriate response because the body has not had enough evolutionary time to cope with modern medicine and organ support. This situation applies equally to the use of nutrition because an injured/infected cave dweller would likely receive little, if any, food and would have to rely on autocannibalism of his/her intrinsic protein and fat stores. Perhaps this may explain the marked loss in body weight and muscle bulk that often occurs during critical illness, despite early and apparently adequate attempts at provision of nutrition.

There are 2 additional points worth making about this hibernatory phase. First, is it triggered by a decrease in energy supply through a combination of direct mitochondrial inhibition and damage, the downregulation of mitochondrial biogenetic processes, and a decreased hormonal stimulation of mitochondrial activity? Alternatively, or perhaps in tandem, is there a primary metabolic switch that reduces energy requirements secondarily? Endogenous delta opioids are implicated in inducing hibernation in bears, so could similar mechanisms exist in humans under prolonged stress?

Second, it is noteworthy that hibernation in response to a prolonged, severe stressor does not guarantee survival, the key to which may lie in the ability to match oxygen supply and demand. This point was demonstrated by higher muscle adenosine triphosphate levels in eventual survivors of septic shock compared with eventual nonsurvivors.[22] In an earlier study, Hayes and colleagues[31] demonstrated that survivors and nonsurvivors of critical illness were clearly identified by their ability (or not) to increase oxygen consumption after inotropic stimulation. Likewise, a study assessing carbon dioxide production as a surrogate of metabolism during sepsis found that death was associated with a lower level of carbon dioxide production.[32] Thus the ability to reduce metabolism seems to be a protective strategy, but this can easily unravel if this reduction is excessive or, alternatively, if it is insufficient to match any primary reduction in energy supply.

THERAPEUTIC IMPLICATIONS AND APPLICATION TO NUTRITION

Accepting that all patients in ICU do not follow a single straight line implies that therapy should be formulated not only to the individual patient but also to match their needs depending on the phase of their illness.

Logically, the early hyperdynamic phase mandates early restoration of organ perfusion not only to minimize the effect of the inflammatory response, which is amplified in the presence of tissue hypoxia, but also to ensure that substrate is adequately delivered to organ beds to service increased cellular needs. On the contrary, the second phase where organ failure is established may benefit from a less aggressive approach. As notable examples, the supranormalization of oxygen delivery through high-dose dobutamine infusion was found to be ineffective[33] or even harmful[31] when administered for a few days to the patients with critical illness. Similarly, administration of growth hormone[34] or thyroxine[35] were significantly detrimental, perhaps because they were given at a point when the body was not ready for them.

Perhaps, nutrition should also mimic these 3 phases, with a high requirement in the first and last phases and a reduced load during the established organ failure (second) phase. Both over- and underfeeding are now recognized as detrimental. Long-term underfeeding increases the risk of nosocomial infection,[36–38] the duration of mechanical ventilation,[39] the length of stay in hospital,[40] and the risk of mortality.[41] On the other hand, overfeeding is deleterious in itself,[42] with parenteral nutrition increasing the susceptibility to complications. Apart from poor glycemic control and its associated morbimortality, increases in nosocomial infection,[43] lipemia, or liver steatosis are well recognized. Furthermore, the effect of under- or overnutrition is not fully elucidated, for example immune modulation. A similar problem exists with immunonutrition. How can one size fit every patient through their critical illness, regardless of whether they are in an immune-stimulated or immune-suppressed state? When stricken by flu, we lose appetite, which is a neurohormonal signal to eat less and decrease substrate intake, and feel fatigued as a direction to work less. When recovering, we become ravenous to meet the surge in the body's metabolic demands.

SUMMARY

In this article, the authors have argued that the body knows intuitively how to cope with the fluctuating course of a critical illness. An early fight may be replaced by a metabolic shutdown in the face of severe, prolonged stress. This shutdown enables survival, preserves longevity, and allows reproduction of individuals with more hardy survival genes. In the recovery phase, or as a prelude to it, energy supplies increase to fuel the anabolic demands leading to an increase in activity. Although this hypothesis lacks definitive confirmation, it does warrant further scrutiny not only in improved timing and titration of therapy but also in modifying the treatment to suit the patient's fluctuating metabolic status, which may include excess intervention. To paraphrase Paracelsus, "everything is poison, it depends on dose."

REFERENCES

1. Martindale RG, McClave SA, Vanek VW, et al. Guidelines for the provision and assessment of nutrition support therapy in the adult critically ill patient: Society of Critical Care Medicine and American Society for Parenteral and Enteral Nutrition. Crit Care Med 2009;37:1757–61.
2. Scurlock C, Mechanick JI. Early nutrition support in the intensive care unit: a US perspective. Curr Opin Clin Nutr Metab Care 2008;11:152–5.
3. Kreymann KG. Early nutrition support in critical care: a European perspective. Curr Opin Clin Nutr Metab Care 2008;11:156–9.
4. Chiolero R, Revelly JP, Tappy L. Energy metabolism in sepsis and injury. Nutrition 1997;13(Suppl 9):45S–51.
5. Jequier E, Acheson K, Schutz Y. Assessment of energy expenditure and fuel utilization in man. Annu Rev Nutr 1987;7:187–208.
6. Kinney JM, Long CL, Gump FE, et al. Tissue composition of weight loss in surgical patients. I. Elective operation. Ann Surg 1968;168:459–74.
7. Weissman C, Kemper M. Assessing hypermetabolism and hypometabolism in the postoperative critically ill patient. Chest 1992;102:1566–71.
8. Kemper M, Weissman C, Hyman AI. Caloric requirements and supply in critically ill surgical patients. Crit Care Med 1992;20:344–8.
9. Brandi LS, Santini L, Bertolini R, et al. Energy expenditure and severity of injury and illness indices in multiple trauma patients. Crit Care Med 1999;27:2684–9.
10. Bruder N, Dumont JC, Francois G. Evolution of energy expenditure and nitrogen excretion in severe head-injured patients. Crit Care Med 1991;19:43–8.
11. Moore R, Najarian MP, Konvolinka CW. Measured energy expenditure in severe head trauma. J Trauma 1989;29:1633–6.
12. Kreymann G, Grosser S, Buggisch P, et al. Oxygen consumption and resting metabolic rate in sepsis, sepsis syndrome, and septic shock. Crit Care Med 1993;21:1012–9.
13. Zauner C, Schuster BI, Schneeweiss B. Similar metabolic responses to standardized total parenteral nutrition of septic and nonseptic critically ill patients. Am J Clin Nutr 2001;74:265–70.

14. McCall M, Jeejeebhoy K, Pencharz P, et al. Effect of neuromuscular blockade on energy expenditure in patients with severe head injury. JPEN J Parenter Enteral Nutr 2003;27:27–35.
15. Hoher JA, Zimermann Teixeira PJ, Hertz F, et al. A comparison between ventilation modes: how does activity level affect energy expenditure estimates? JPEN J Parenter Enteral Nutr 2008;32:176–83.
16. Jeevanandam M, Young DH, Schiller WR. Obesity and the metabolic response to severe multiple trauma in man. J Clin Invest 1991;87:262–9.
17. Watters JM, Redmond ML, Desai D, et al. Effects of age and body composition on the metabolic responses to elective colon resection. Ann Surg 1990;212:213–20.
18. Van den Berghe G. Novel insights into the neuroendocrinology of critical illness. Eur J Endocrinol 2000;143:1–13.
19. Reid CL, Campbell IT, Little RA. Muscle wasting and energy balance in critical illness. Clin Nutr 2004;23:273–80.
20. Soop A, Albert J, Weitzberg E, et al. Complement activation, endothelin-1 and neuropeptide Y in relation to the cardiovascular response to endotoxin-induced systemic inflammation in healthy volunteers. Acta Anaesthesiol Scand 2004;48:74–81.
21. Hotchkiss RS, Karl IE. The pathophysiology and treatment of sepsis. N Engl J Med 2003;348:138–50.
22. Brealey D, Brand M, Hargreaves I, et al. Association between mitochondrial dysfunction and severity and outcome of septic shock. Lancet 2002;360:219–23.
23. Hotchkiss RS, Tinsley KW, Swanson PE, et al. Endothelial cell apoptosis in sepsis. Crit Care Med 2002;30(Suppl 5):S225–8.
24. Hotchkiss RS, Swanson PE, Freeman BD, et al. Apoptotic cell death in patients with sepsis, shock, and multiple organ dysfunction. Crit Care Med 1999;27:1230–51.
25. Levy RJ, Piel DA, Acton PD, et al. Evidence of myocardial hibernation in the septic heart. Crit Care Med 2005;33:2752–6.
26. Schiffl H, Fischer R. Five-year outcomes of severe acute kidney injury requiring renal replacement therapy. Nephrol Dial Transplant 2008;23:2235–41.
27. Wan L, Bagshaw SM, Langenberg C, et al. Pathophysiology of septic acute kidney injury: what do we really know? Crit Care Med 2008;36(4 Suppl):S198–203.
28. Boekstegers P, Weidenhofer S, Kapsner T, et al. Skeletal muscle partial pressure of oxygen in patients with sepsis. Crit Care Med 1994;22:640–50.
29. Singer M, De Santis V, Vitale D, et al. Multiorgan failure is an adaptive, endocrine-mediated, metabolic response to overwhelming systemic inflammation. Lancet 2004;364:545–8.
30. Mongardon N, Dyson A, Singer M. Is MOF an outcome parameter or a transient, adaptive state in critical illness? Curr Opin Crit Care 2009;15:431–6.
31. Hayes MA, Timmins AC, Yau EH, et al. Elevation of systemic oxygen delivery in the treatment of critically ill patients. N Engl J Med 1994;330:1717–22.
32. Kao CC, Guntupalli KK, Bandi V, et al. Whole-body CO_2 production as an index of the metabolic response to sepsis. Shock 2009;32:23–8.
33. Gattinoni L, Brazzi L, Pelosi P, et al. A trial of goal-oriented hemodynamic therapy in critically ill patients. SvO2 Collaborative Group. N Engl J Med 1995;333:1025–32.
34. Takala J, Ruokonen E, Webster NR, et al. Increased mortality associated with growth hormone treatment in critically ill adults. N Engl J Med 1999;341:785–92.
35. Acker CG, Singh AR, Flick RP, et al. A trial of thyroxine in acute renal failure. Kidney Int 2000;57:293–8.

36. Dvir D, Cohen J, Singer P. Computerized energy balance and complications in critically ill patients: an observational study. Clin Nutr 2006;25:37–44.
37. Rubinson L, Diette GB, Song X, et al. Low caloric intake is associated with nosocomial bloodstream infections in patients in the medical intensive care unit. Crit Care Med 2004;32:350-7.
38. Villet S, Chiolero RL, Bollmann MD, et al. Negative impact of hypocaloric feeding and energy balance on clinical outcome in ICU patients. Clin Nutr 2005;24:502–9.
39. Barr J, Hecht M, Flavin KE, et al. Outcomes in critically ill patients before and after the implementation of an evidence-based nutritional management protocol. Chest 2004;125:1446–57.
40. Martin CM, Doig GS, Heyland DK, et al. Multicenter, cluster-randomized clinical trial of algorithms for critical-care enteral and parenteral therapy (ACCEPT). CMAJ 2004;170:197–204.
41. Faisy C, Lerolle N, Dachraoui F, et al. Impact of energy deficit calculated by a predictive method on outcome in medical patients requiring prolonged acute mechanical ventilation. Br J Nutr 2009;101:1079–87.
42. Griffiths RD. Too much of a good thing: the curse of overfeeding. Crit Care 2007; 11:176.
43. Dissanaike S, Shelton M, Warner K, et al. The risk for bloodstream infections is associated with increased parenteral caloric intake in patients receiving parenteral nutrition. Crit Care 2007;11:R114.

Clinical Guidelines and Nutrition Therapy: Better Understanding and Greater Application to Patient Care

Stephen A. McClave, MD[a],*, Ryan T. Hurt, MD[b,c,d]

KEYWORDS

• Guidelines • Parenteral nutrition • Enteral nutrition • Mortality

Clinical guidelines are essentially recommendations for patient care based on the best available data. These guidelines are not absolute requirements, do not guarantee outcome or mortality benefits, and are certainly never a substitute for clinical judgment. In fact, at the bedside, clinical judgment always takes precedence over any societal guidelines. Nonetheless, clinical guidelines developed by medical specialty and subspecialty societies are some of the more rigorously supported documents in the literature. The current emphasis on evidence-based medicine mandates that guidelines be supported by current literature. Although the focus lies primarily on prospective randomized controlled trials (PRCTs), most guideline committees review other national and international societal guidelines and at times, include expert opinion or consensus recommendations. It is important that guidelines should have clinical practicality and should promote knowledge translation where the evidence in the literature ultimately relegates directly to patient care.

However, the explosion of guidelines in the literature can be frustrating for the clinician. Guidelines between societies often contradict each other, and certain guidelines often contradict practice at individual institutions. However, controversy offers an

[a] Division of Gastroenterology, Hepatology and Nutrition, Department of Medicine, University of Louisville School of Medicine, 550 South Jackson Street, Louisville, KY 40202, USA
[b] Division of General Internal Medicine, Mayo Clinic, 200 1st Street SW, Rochester, MN 55905, USA
[c] Department of Medicine, University of Louisville School of Medicine, Louisville, KY, USA
[d] Department of Physiology and Biophysics, University of Louisville School of Medicine, Louisville, KY, USA
* Corresponding author.
E-mail address: Stephen.McClave@louisville.edu

Crit Care Clin 26 (2010) 451–466
doi:10.1016/j.ccc.2010.04.008   criticalcare.theclinics.com
0749-0704/10/$ – see front matter © 2010 Elsevier Inc. All rights reserved.

opportunity for growth. The most important aspect of a good clinical guideline is transparency, that is, there should be a direct connection between the clinical recommendation and the underlying studies from which it gets its support. Identifying areas of controversy, seeking out the underlying studies, and determining individual interpretation of the studies should lead to the decision of whether or not to change clinical practice.

DERIVATION OF THE SOCIETY OF CRITICAL CARE MEDICINE/AMERICAN SOCIETY FOR PARENTERAL AND ENTERAL NUTRITION 2009 GUIDELINES

The predecessor for the Society of Critical Care Medicine (SCCM)/American Society for Parenteral and Enteral Nutrition (A.S.P.E.N.) guidelines[1] was the 2002 A.S.P.E.N. Critical Care Guidelines.[2] The development of these guidelines was a huge project for A.S.P.E.N., which included guidelines for nutrition therapy across a wide variety of patient populations and clinical scenarios. These guidelines were published in an older format, in which there were 3 or 4 pages of text followed by only 4 generalized recommendations. In July 2004, a guideline committee was requested to revise the critical care guidelines published in 2002. The original manuscript was written in the old style and submitted for review in July 2005.

However, as this committee was developing these revised guidelines, the overall landscape for clinical guidelines was already changing. In 2003, the Canadian Critical Care Group under the direction of Daren Hyland published the "Canadian clinical practice guidelines for nutrition support in mechanically ventilated, critically ill adult patients."[3] This publication was followed a year later by a multisociety task force publication entitled "Surviving sepsis campaign guidelines for management of severe sepsis and septic shock."[4] Both of these publications altered the format for societal guidelines. In contrast to the old style with long text and minimally brief generalized recommendations, the new style of these 2 publications was topic driven, brief, clear, and very specific. A particular clinical recommendation was followed by a brief discussion, which promoted transparency between the clinical guideline statement and the underlying supportive evidence. In addition, the guidelines were renewable and were freely accessible to the public (not simply reserved for societal members).

As a result of the changes in the overall landscape of guidelines, a voluntary revision of the A.S.P.E.N. Critical Care Guidelines was made and resubmitted a year later in 2006. At some point in the process, a decision was made that the guidelines should be a joint project between SCCM and A.S.P.E.N. The 2 guideline committees were merged, and all subsequent revisions of the manuscript were a joint effort by these 2 societies and this single combined committee. The committee was composed of critical care surgeons, gastroenterologists, nurses, and dietitians. Although 2 pharmacists were named to the original committee, they had little input into the final recommendations that were ultimately published.

Overall, the publication of guidelines involved a 5-year process from July 2004 to the final approval in January 2009. There were 5 full rounds of review, with more than 50 reviewers interpreting the manuscript, and the final approval was required from 3 separate boards (the A.S.P.E.N. Board of Directors, the SCCM Council, and the American College of Critical Care Medicine Board of Regents). The final guidelines were published in full text in the *Journal of Parenteral and Enteral Nutrition (JPEN)* in the May 2009 issue,[1] with an executive summary being published in the same month in the journal *Critical Care Medicine*.[5]

The process of development of guidelines began with the committee compiling a list of recommendations or action statements. The committee then referred to the literature focusing on PRCTs as the primary source for support. The overall strength for a particular recommendation was based on 2 things: the level of the investigative studies and the number of studies that supported that particular recommendation. Controversy in interpreting the literature was resolved by consensus opinion of the committee members. However, for certain issues, the committee members actually downgraded the final recommendation out of respect for an opposing opinion. The philosophy of this particular committee was that they decided to include patient care recommendations even when the sole basis of support was expert opinion. It was clear on review of the literature that many aspects of clinical practice in nutrition therapy were not supported by PRCTs. In a lengthy process, such as the derivation of guidelines, in which so many expert reviewers would be involved, the committee saw a unique opportunity to derive guidelines even though support from the literature was solely based on expert opinion. The committee was also acutely aware of the polarity in the critical care community with regard to use of parenteral nutrition (PN) in the intensive care unit (ICU). Therefore, the committee decided that it was most important to provide specific recommendations for the use of PN, identifying those conditions in particular patients in whom outcome benefit could be assured with the use of PN.

One of the early areas of controversy was in the definition of a large clinical trial. Any study that performed a formal power analysis, identified endpoint criteria, and then continued to enroll enough patients to meet those criteria was considered a large trial (in which the chances for alpha and beta errors were minimized). But most studies in the literature that dated more than 5 years from their date of publication did not have a power analysis. It was decided that an arbitrary number of more than 100 subjects would define a large study in the absence of a power analysis.

Another controversy that existed for the guideline committee was the use of meta-analysis. Some societal guidelines have used meta-analysis as the highest grade of literature. The SCCM/A.S.P.E.N. Guidelines Committee, however, thought that meta-analysis should be used to help organize information and derive a treatment effect from multiple trials but should not be used to grade the overall strength of the recommendation. The ultimate grade for the recommendation had to be based on the level of evidence of the individual studies. Review articles or consensus statements from expert panels were considered as expert opinion and given the lowest level of grading strength.

Despite the structured format followed by the Guidelines Committee and the extensive review by more than 50 experts and 3 societal boards of directors, there were still areas of intense controversy that made derivation of the final recommendations extremely difficult. The following are several examples of controversy, based on the literature itself, the perspective taken by the SCCM/A.S.P.E.N. Guidelines Committee, or the clinical implications of the recommendations that immediately followed publication.

Permissive Underfeeding in the Morbidly Obese Critically Ill Patient

In the section on dosing of enteral feeding, the SCCM/A.S.P.E.N. guidelines recommended that in the critically ill obese patient, permissive underfeeding with enteral nutrition (EN) should be considered.[1] For all classes of obesity (in which the body mass index [BMI] calculated as the weight in kilograms divided by height in meters squared is >30), the goal of the enteral feeding regimen should be to provide 60% to 70% of target caloric requirements. These caloric requirements could be identified by simple weight-based equations such as 11 to 14 kcal/kg actual body weight

(ABW)/d, or 22 to 25 kcal/kg ideal body weight (IBW)/d. Certainly, the use of indirect calorimetry provides a more accurate measure of caloric requirements, and setting the goal of feeding at 60% to 70% of the measured resting energy expenditure would be appropriate for permissive underfeeding. Protein requirements were slightly more complicated, such that for patients with class I and class II obesity with a BMI of 30 to 40, 2.0 g protein/kg IBW/d should be provided, whereas for patients with class III obesity and a BMI greater than 40, more than 2.6 g protein/kg IBW/d should be provided. The strength of these recommendations was grade D, based on retrospective data with historical controls. A report by Choban and Dickerson[6] showed that 2.0 g/kg IBW/d of protein is required for patients with class I and II obesity to reach nitrogen balance, whereas more than 2.6 g/kg IBW/d of protein is required for an obese patient with a BMI greater than 40. However, there are virtually no data to define how much of protein is required for the superobese patients with BMI greater than 50.

Controversial reports from the literature provide information that obesity may be a benefit in the ICU setting, contradicting the rationale for permissive underfeeding. When critically ill obese patients in a surgical or medical ICU are compared with lean controls, obesity is associated with increased infection, ICU and hospital length of stay, multiple organ failure, and duration on mechanical ventilation.[7,8] For reasons that are not entirely clear, mortality is increased in trauma patients in a surgical ICU, whereas mortality is decreased in obese patients in a medical ICU compared with lean controls.[7,8] This observation has led pulmonary critical care clinicians managing patients in a medical ICU to see obesity as a benefit in critical illness, that is, excess fuel stores protect the patient and improve survival. A report by Alberda and colleagues,[9] involving an international survey of ICUs around the world, showed that patients with a BMI greater than 30 showed a reduced mortality when an extra 1000 cal was provided in their nutrition regimen. The concepts presented by these articles would suggest that in the critical care setting permissive underfeeding might have deleterious effects, even in obesity.

Resolving this controversy can be very difficult for the individual practitioner. At the authors' institution, they reviewed the effect of morbid obesity and its interference with virtually every aspect of patient care. Special equipment is required with big boy beds, wheelchairs, and toilet seats. It is difficult to turn the patients adequately, which increases the chances for pressure sores, atelectasis, and pneumonia. The morbidly obese patient presents a risk to health care providers. Obese patients are difficult to ventilate and are prone to sleep apnea and restrictive lung disease. Development of complications is difficult to evaluate because of difficulties in transporting and performing diagnostic tests in morbidly obese patients. The failure to ambulate these patients adequately increases the risk for deep venous thrombosis. Underlying hepatobiliary diseases, such as nonalcoholic steatohepatitis and cirrhosis, and the respiratory abnormalities from obstructive sleep apnea and restrictive lung disease promote multiple organ failure.

Older physiologic studies from the past would suggest that as long as adequate protein is provided, calories can be restricted, the fat mass can be reduced, and the lean body mass can be maintained. In a study by Elwyn,[10] reducing the energy intake as a percentage of energy expenditure to less than 60% still resulted in neutral or even positive nitrogen balance as long as the protein intake was increased to 2.2 g/kg/d. In a subsequent study by Hill and Church,[11] total caloric energy intake could be reduced to as low as 20 kcal/kg/d and the body fat mass could be reduced successfully. By increasing the nitrogen uptake from 0.9 to as high as 2.2 g/kg/d of protein, erosion of the lean body mass could be prevented.[11]

From these physiologic studies and the adverse effect of morbid obesity on every aspect of patient care, the authors' institution interpreted the guideline recommendation for permissive underfeeding of the morbidly obese critically ill patient to be appropriate as long as adequate protein delivery is provided.

The Effect of Protocols for Gastric Residual Volumes on Tolerance of EN

In the section on tolerance of EN, the SCCM/A.S.P.E.N. guidelines recommended that evidence for bowel motility and resolution of ileus was not required before initiation of enteral feeding.[1] But as enteral feeding is started, the patient should be monitored for tolerance. The guidelines recommend avoiding inappropriate cessation of enteral feeding, minimizing periods during which patients were kept nil per os for tests or procedures (to avoid prolonged ileus), and avoiding holding EN for gastric residual volumes less than 500 mL in the absence of other signs of intolerance.[1]

Recommending that the cutoff value for gastric residual volume be raised to 500 mL was incredibly controversial. This recommendation, however, was based on 3 level 2 (small randomized)[12–14] trials and 1 level 1 (large randomized)[15] trial. In each study, patients were randomized to 2 different cutoff values for the gastric residual volume and adverse patient outcome, such as regurgitation, vomiting, aspiration, or overall complications, was less in the group randomized to the higher cutoff value for residual volume (reaching significance in 2 of the studies).[12,15] By raising the cutoff value for the gastric residual volume, 2 of the studies demonstrated that patients received a significantly higher volume of EN.[12,15] Two more prospective trials compared routine checking of residual volumes with no checking of gastric residual volumes.[16,17] In the study by Powell and colleagues,[16] incidence of aspiration pneumonia was not significantly different between the 2 groups but tube clogging was reduced 10-fold in the group for which no residual volumes were monitored. In the study by Reignier and colleagues,[17] which was performed prospectively before and after the implementation of a protocol, the group for which no residual volumes were measured had less-frequent evidence of intolerance, received a greater volume of enteral feeding that was infused, and had no difference in the incidence of vomiting or ventilator-associated pneumonia when compared with the group for which residual volumes were measured routinely. To better interpret the SCCM/A.S.P.E.N. guidelines,[1] it is important to note that increasing the volume of EN delivered often decreases the incidence of pneumonia. Thus, lowering the gastric residual volume to protect the patient may impede EN delivery and the risk of pneumonia may actually increase. In a study by Meissner and colleagues,[18] the narcotic antagonist, naloxone, was infused through the tube by enteral feeding in study patients, whereas controls received enteral feeding alone. This strategy, which reversed the effects of systemic analgesia at the level of the gut, succeeded in significantly increasing the amount of EN infused. As a result, the incidence of pneumonia was decreased significantly from 55% in study patients to 36% in controls ($P<.05$).[18] In a study by Kudsk and colleagues[19] on trauma patients, those who received enteral feeding had a 3-fold reduction in pneumonia compared with those randomized to PN. Again, in the study by Taylor and colleagues,[12] use of an aggressive protocol with high gastric residual volumes in study patients succeeded in nearly doubling the percentage of goal calories infused compared with a more conservative protocol with lower gastric residual volumes in controls, and as a result the incidence of pneumonia was reduced from 63% to 44%, respectively (P = not significant [NS]).

Thus, although the recommendation of SCCM/A.S.P.E.N. to raise the cutoff value for gastric residual volume to 500 mL was highly controversial,[1] the recommendation is very well supported in the literature.

Use of Pharmaconutrition Formulas

Out of 76 total recommendations, only 2 guideline statements in the SCCM/A.S.P.E.N. guidelines were given a grade A recommendation.[1] For surgical ICUs, the recommendation that immune-modulating enteral formulations supplemented with agents such as arginine, glutamine, ω-3 fatty acids, and antioxidants should be used for major elective surgery was given a grade A. However, the use of arginine-containing pharmaconutrient formulas in the general ICU population was much more controversial. A meta-analysis by Heyland and Novak[20] in 2001, a report by Bower and colleagues,[21] and a study by Dent published only in abstract form[22] showed a higher mortality in patients receiving an arginine-containing immune formula compared with controls receiving a standard formula. Patients who received the arginine-containing formula had a mortality of 15.7%, which was significantly greater than controls with a mortality of 8.4% ($P = .055$).[21] The difference in mortality rate was even greater in those patients who died as a direct result of sepsis. This study was criticized for having a possible error of randomization, because the Acute Physiology and Chronic Health Evaluation (APACHE) II score in patients who died in the immune group was 19.2 ± 5.6, which was significantly greater than the mean APACHE II score of 12.7 ± 2.1 in patients who died in the control group ($P<.05$).[21] However, this criticism is an error because the APACHE II scores on admission were not significantly different between study patients and controls (15.9 ± 5.4 vs 15.6 ± 4.8, respectively, $P = $ NS).[21]

In the Ross unpublished study, patients who received an arginine-containing formula had a mortality rate of 23.0%, which was significantly greater than that seen in controls at 9.6% ($P = .03$).[22] However, this study was thought to have an error in randomization. Out of 35 elderly patients with pneumonia, 26 were included in the study group receiving the arginine formula. Half of the deaths in the immune group were attributed to this elderly population with preexisting pneumonia. The study was also criticized because the formula used for this study, Optimental (Abbott Nutrition Inc, Columbus, OH, USA), had only one-third the content of arginine in another formula, Impact (Nestlé Healthcare Nutrition Inc, Gland, Switzerland), that was used in previous studies.[22] A third study by Bertolini and colleagues[23] had an odd design in which an immune-modulating arginine-containing enteral formula was compared with PN. Although ICU mortality was significantly greater in the group that received the arginine-containing enteral formula when compared with controls receiving PN (44.4% vs 14.3%, respectively, $P = .039$), the 28-day mortality and overall hospital mortality were not significantly different between groups.[23]

A study by Galban and colleagues[24] was performed in a critically ill population in which 100% of patients had sepsis and the opposite results were found. Study patients receiving an arginine-containing formula had a significantly lower mortality than controls receiving a standard enteral formula (19.1% vs 32.2%, respectively, $P<.05$).[24] Mortality directly related to infection was also significantly less in the group receiving the arginine formula compared with controls (14.6% vs 26.4%, respectively, $P = .05$).[24] Heyland and Novak[20] criticized this study because the mortality effect was seen only in those patients with an APACHE II score of 10 to 15. With higher APACHE II scores, the benefit effect lost significance. This criticism of the study by Galban and colleagues[24] may not be fair, in that the study was powered to show a difference in overall mortality between the study group and controls and not powered to look at a subset of mortality between groups for different ranges of the APACHE II score.

This controversy made it difficult for the SCCM/A.S.P.E.N. Guidelines Committee to make their recommendations regarding the use of arginine formulas in the ICU population. When the guidelines were being developed, a large study by Kieft and colleagues[25] showed absolutely no difference in patient outcome between the study group that received an arginine-containing formula and controls that received a standard enteral formula with regard to mortality, infection, hospital length of stay, and duration of mechanical ventilation. When the committee analyzed the revised updated Canadian clinical practice guidelines' meta-analysis on use of arginine-containing formulas,[26] it was found that the ICU length of stay was still significantly reduced by 0.36 days ($P = .50$), hospital length of stay was reduced by 0.33 days (an effect which just missed significance, $P = .06$), and duration of mechanical ventilation was reduced by 0.30 days ($P = .09$) compared with use of standard enteral formulations.[26] The Canadian Clinical Practice Guideline Committee interpreted this literature in such a way as to recommend that arginine-containing formulas not be used in the patient in medical ICU.[3] The Evidence Analysis Library created by the American Dietetic Association made no recommendation on the use of arginine-containing formulas because of the controversy.[27] However, the SCCM/A.S.P.E.N. Guidelines Committee interpreted this literature in such a way that the use of an arginine-containing formula in a surgical ICU was given a grade A recommendation, whereas the use of an arginine-containing formula in a medical ICU was given a grade B recommendation.[1]

To further complicate an already strong controversy, Luiking and colleagues[28] performed studies in which arginine was infused directly into the systemic circulation of septic medical and surgical patients. Results showed no evidence of hemodynamic compromise with the administration of arginine comparable to the doses seen with the provision of enteral pharmaconutrition formulas. Another issue complicating this controversy involves asymmetric dimethylarginine (ADMA), an agent that competes with L-arginine for production of inducible nitric oxide synthetase (iNOS). L-Arginine stimulates iNOS production and results in a clinical effect of vasodilation, stimulation of host defense, and perfusion of tissue. ADMA has the opposite effect, inhibiting iNOS production, causing vasoconstriction, and reducing tissue perfusion. In a large study of patients with critical illness, ADMA levels were shown to be elevated, correlating with increased ICU length of stay, multiple organ failure, and mortality.[29] Response to infusion of L-arginine was predicated by the levels of ADMA and the balance between these 2 agents.[30] In a normal setting, the volume of L-arginine is greater than ADMA in the systemic circulation and as a result, nitric oxide synthetase is induced and vasodilation occurs. However, when an excess of ADMA accumulates, iNOS production is inhibited, less nitric oxide is produced, and vasoconstriction occurs. Providing L-arginine reverses the effects of ADMA, restores balance between the 2 agents, and promotes vasodilation, tissue perfusion, and protection of endothelial function.[29,30]

With a controversy of this degree, there may be no correct answer. The SCCM/A.S.P.E.N. Guidelines Committee was careful to base their recommendations on the strength of the literature, acknowledge the controversy, and downgrade the recommendation for use of arginine-containing pharmaconutrient formulas in the patient in medical ICU (adding a provision that use in severely septic patients should be done with caution).[1] Individual practitioners are encouraged to review the literature themselves to determine institutional policy.

Safety of Fish Oil

The only other grade A recommendation out of the 76 guideline statements published in the SCCM/A.S.P.E.N. guidelines involved the use of fish oil in patients with respiratory failure.[1] The recommendation specifically stated that patients with acute respiratory distress syndrome (ARDS) and severe acute lung injury should be placed on an enteral formula characterized by an antiinflammatory lipid profile (eg, ω-3 fish oils, borage oil) and antioxidants.[1] Within months of the publication of this recommendation, the safety of fish oil was called into question because of the cessation of a grant through the National Heart, Lung, and Blood Institute (NHLBI) involving the ARDS clinical network (ARDSNet) group.[31] The ARDSNet group is a pulmonary critical care NHLBI-sponsored study group that has performed excellent studies in critical care for the past 10 to 15 years. In the summer of 2009, a portion of the EDEN-Omega study by this group was terminated for reasons of futility.[31] The study was originally of a 2 × 2 × 2 design, involving a bronchodilator versus placebo, trophic feeds (ramp-up slowly over several days) versus full feeds (reach the goal within 24 hours), and a fish oil/borage oil supplement versus placebo. The fish oil/borage oil supplement was designed by Abbott Nutrition Inc to replicate the ingredients in the commercial product Oxepa. However, instead of being infused continuously as part of the enteral formula, the supplement was given as a bolus twice a day separated from the enteral formula. Controls received a placebo that was composed of a formula with none of the active ingredients of the antiinflammatory lipids or antioxidants. Halfway through the study, at the interim analysis,[31] the study was stopped for reasons of futility and not for ethical reasons. Although nothing has been formally published so far, communication with the primary investigators indicated that the control group had a very low mortality rate, which was far less than that seen in the controls from any of the other studies involving the ARDSNet group (Todd Rice, MD, Personal communication, 2009). The study group receiving the fish oil/borage oil supplement had a higher mortality. Halfway through the study, it seemed that there was no chance, regardless of the value of the supplement, for the study patients to catch up with the controls in regard to mortality. Had there been a clear signal of danger, it would have mandated that the study be stopped for ethical reasons. Another interpretation expressed by the investigators was that the supplement seemed to have no effect, raising concern that the bolus infusion resulted in simple catabolism and breakdown of the supplement without use (Todd Rice, MD, Personal communication, 2009). It is also possible that bolus dosing of a large dose of fish oil to the gut of a critically ill patient leads to malabsorption of the fat and this contributes to lack of efficacy. The controversy surrounding this issue is related to whether the difference in mortality rates raised a danger signal that would contradict the original recommendation in the SCCM/A.S.P.E.N. guidelines. Little data exist elsewhere in the literature to suggest an adverse effect from fish oil, and communication expressed by the investigators of the Omega arm of the EDEN-Omega study up to this point indicates that they do not think there is any signal of harm involved with fish oil use in ARDS.

Use of Supplemental PN

One of the most controversial areas of the SCCM/A.S.P.E.N. guidelines was the recommendations for the use of supplemental PN in a patient already receiving EN. In the section regarding dosing of EN, recommendations were made to provide more than 50% to 65% of goal calories during the first week to achieve the clinical benefits of EN (grade C recommendation).[1] Further recommendations were to add supplemental PN only if provision of EN alone was unable to meet goal calorie requirements after 7 to 10 days (grade E recommendation). Adding PN before 7 to 10 days did not seem to improve outcome and might increase risk to the patient (grade C recommendation).[1] This recommendation was one of many by the Guidelines Committee to minimize the polarity involved with the use of PN in the ICU. The recommendation for use of supplemental PN was based on 5 PRCTs of EN alone versus EN supplemented with PN[32–36] and a meta-analysis by Heyland and colleagues[3] published in 2003. The meta-analysis showed significantly greater cost and a trend toward greater mortality when EN was supplemented with PN and no difference in infection, hospital length of stay, or duration of mechanical ventilation in patients in whom EN was supplemented with PN when compared with patients receiving EN alone.[3] In a study in burn patients, there was evidence of immune suppression when PN was added to EN, and the mortality increased from 26% in patients receiving EN alone to 63% in patients receiving EN supplemented with PN ($P<.05$).[32]

These recommendations for use of PN were highly controversial in that they contradicted practice and recommendation of the European nutrition community and the European Society for Parenteral and Enteral Nutrition (ESPEN) guidelines. A very important study by Villet and colleagues[37] evaluated the concept of cumulative caloric deficit, showing that patients in ICU accrue an energy deficit because ongoing energy expenditure is not met by caloric provision due to delays in delivery of nutrition therapy. The cumulative energy deficit in this study was shown to correlate with the increased hospital length of stay, infections, overall complications, and duration of mechanical ventilation (all endpoints $P<.04$).[37] As a result of this study and others, the ESPEN recommended supplementing EN with PN if, by 24 hours, more than 80% of energy requirements are not met by EN alone.[38]

Again, in a controversy of this nature, there seems to be no correct answer based on the available literature. Studies support and refute the recommendation provided by the SCCM/A.S.P.E.N. Guidelines Committee. The Glue Grant study was a large multicenter trial, which evaluated severely injured trauma patients and use of PN.[39] Data were gathered prospectively and then reviewed retrospectively in 567 trauma patients, of whom 17% received PN only, 87% received EN only, and 13% received a combination of both. Results showed that any use of PN was associated with an increased risk of infection ($P<.01$). Mortality was higher in patients who received EN supplemented with PN when compared with those receiving EN alone ($P<.06$).[39] A second national prospective observational study of similar design from Germany studied the same issues in 415 patients with severe sepsis or septic shock.[40] Again, 20.1% received EN alone, 35.1% received PN alone, and the remaining 34.6% received a combination of both. Exclusive use of PN was associated with the highest mortality at 62.3%, whereas the mortality with the use of EN only was lowest at 38.9% (the difference being statistically significant, $P<.005$).[40] Even when adjusted for comorbidities, use of PN was still predictive of increased mortality. In a study similar to that of Villet and colleagues',[37] Dvir and colleagues[41] also looked at cumulative energy deficit. The investigators showed that a negative cumulative caloric deficit correlated significantly with ARDS, sepsis, renal failure, pressure sores, need for surgery, and total complications ($P<.02$ for all outcome effects), whereas there was no correlation to ICU or hospital length of stay, duration of mechanical ventilation, or mortality.[41]

The criticism of these studies relates to the fact that because they were nonrandomized, patients receiving EN alone may not have been as sick as those who were underfed by the enteral route and thus had to be supplemented by PN. Therefore, it is difficult to resolve this particular controversy based on the literature that is available at present. Four large international research groups have designed and initiated similar studies evaluating hospitalized patients randomized to EN alone versus EN supplemented with PN soon after their admission. The primary investigators for these research groups include Greet Van den Berghe, Daren Heyland, Claude Pichardc, and Gordon Doig. Hopefully, any one of these large, well-designed studies should provide valuable data to help resolve the seemingly contradictory recommendations from the ESPEN and SCCM/A.S.P.E.N. guidelines regarding use of supplemental PN in the ICU.[1,38]

EFFECT OF GUIDELINES ON PATIENT OUTCOME

The manner in which guidelines are derived at present implies that recommendations supported by evidence-based medicine should result in better patient care. Early data addressing this question have shown a lack of effect from use of such societal guidelines. A study by Jain and colleagues[42] using cluster randomization assigned medical centers to active dissemination of the Canadian clinical practice guidelines (which involved education, training, and feedback on the guidelines) or passive dissemination (which involved only receipt of the guidelines). At the end of the study there were no significant differences in adequacy of EN delivery, mortality, hospital length of stay, or ICU length of stay between the 2 groups. The only benefit from active dissemination of the guidelines (compared with passive) was improved glycemic control.[42] In a study of similar design, Doig and colleagues[43] prospectively evaluated patients in medical centers who were randomized to aggressive use of the Australian/New Zealand guidelines versus controls who were delivered nutrition support without the benefit of the guidelines. A slight but significant improvement in the time to initiate EN was seen in the guideline study group compared with controls (0.75 days vs 1.37 days, respectively, $P<.05$). However, mortality, hospital length of stay, and ICU length of stay were not different between the 2 groups.[43]

The negative results from these 2 studies would suggest that guidelines have little effect on patient outcome. However, most studies were performed immediately after a period of intense study and development of guidelines for each of the national groups in those countries. In both the studies, the control group received early, effective, adequate nutritional therapy.[42,43] It may have been nearly impossible for the study groups, regardless of the quality or efficacy of the guidelines, to improve on the excellent nutrition therapy delivered to controls. The lack of response, however, does raise questions about barriers to delivery of nutrition therapy, whether guidelines successfully equate to practical bedside action statements, or whether guidelines have to be translated into clinical pathways, nurse-driven protocols, or physician orders to be effective.

DO GUIDELINES OVERLY RELY ON EVIDENCE-BASED MEDICINE AND PRCTS?

After more than a decade of emphasis on evidence-based medicine and the mandate that clinical practice should be supported by the highest level of clinical research, a controversy has arisen over the reliance of guidelines solely on PRCTs. For the SCCM/A.S.P.E.N. guidelines, any A, B, or C grade recommendation had to be supported by PRCTs.[1] Recommendations based on expert opinion or studies with historical or concurrent nonrandomized controls were relegated to grade D or E. More than 60% of the SCCM/A.S.P.E.N. recommendations were A, B, or C grade recommendations and were based on PRCTs.[1] The Canadian practice guidelines use only PRCTs in the derivation of their guidelines.[3] Several major societies such as the World Health Organization, SCCM, A.S.P.E.N., and The Endocrine Society have adapted the grading of recommendations, assessment, development, and evaluation (GRADE) system, formulated by the GRADE working group, for creating guidelines.[44] This system is designed to add structured subjectivity to interpretation of the PRCTs from the literature. The GRADE system starts by evaluating and ranking individual studies from the highest grade at 4+ to the lowest at 1+ and then applies several subjective qualifiers.[44] The qualifiers include methodological quality, magnitude of the treatment effect, precision estimate of the treatment effect, outcome importance, risk of therapy, resource use, and varying other subjective values that may be deemed important by the Guidelines Committee. Based on the strength of the original study and the filter of the subjective qualifiers, the final guideline statement is then rated as either a strong recommendation (desirable effects outweigh the undesirable effects) or a weak recommendation (recommendation is suggested with the knowledge that desirable effects probably outweigh the undesirable effects).[44]

A recent letter to the *JPEN* editor in response to the SCCM/A.S.P.E.N. guidelines demonstrates some of the difficulties that could arise when a guideline committee interprets clinical studies through the filter of subjective qualifiers.[45] In the letter to the editor, Bistrian[45] refuted the SCCM/A.S.P.E.N. recommendation that EN should be used preferentially over PN in the critically ill patient. Bistrian argued that the opposite is true, that is, PN should be preferred over EN, based on the meta-analysis by Simpson and Doig[46] showing that there was lower mortality with PN compared with EN. He thought that there was less bias in this meta-analysis because of the emphasis on intent-to-treat basis, despite the fact that the results of this meta-analysis were exactly opposite to that of 4 other meta-analyses by Gramlich and colleagues,[47] Moore and colleagues,[48] Peter and colleagues,[49] and Heyland and colleagues.[50] In the introduction of the meta-analysis by Simpson and Doig,[46] the investigators discussed methodological quality and the importance of 3 key components: intent-to-treat analysis, concealed randomization, and appropriate use of blinding. Applying a subjective filter (based on these methodological components) to their selection of studies for the meta-analysis, the investigators ended up aggregating the data from 9 studies. Results showed a reduced mortality with use of PN compared with EN in critically ill patients. The meta-analysis also showed that infectious morbidity was worse with PN than with EN. Yet the investigators made no attempt to provide an explanation for the differential effect on mortality.[46]

The treatment effect of PN on mortality in this meta-analysis was driven specifically by 2 studies conducted by Rapp and colleagues[51] and Woodcock and colleagues.[52] Although the study by Woodcock and colleagues[52] was large, including a total of 562 patients, only 11.4% were actually randomized to EN or PN. The mortality was lower in the PN group than in the EN group but the difference did not reach statistical significance. The report by Rapp and colleagues[51] was the first of 3 studies performed by a neurosurgery group from the University of Kentucky evaluating EN versus PN in trauma patients with head injury. This initial study conducted in 1983 showed a significantly lower mortality in the PN group compared with the EN group (0% vs 44%, respectively, $P<.05$).[51] However, although the study design was described by Simpson and Doig[46] as a comparison between early PN and early EN, controls really received standard therapy or no nutritional support (patients were on their own to advance to oral feeding).[51] In subsequent publications, this research group from the University of Kentucky referred to the controls from this study as undergoing starvation.[53] The second study published 4 years later, again in trauma patients with head injury, compared early PN with early EN (this time EN was delivered by infusion into the stomach via a nasogastric tube).[53] The frequency of a favorable outcome based on recovery of neurologic injury was significantly higher at the 3-month mark in the PN group compared with controls receiving EN (43.5% vs 17.9%, respectively, $P<.05$).[53] Mortality was actually higher in the PN study group than in the controls (43.5% vs 35.7%, respectively, $P = NS$).[53] This same research group published a third study in 1994 (in abstract form only), in which trauma patients were randomized to 1 of 3 groups: early PN, standard therapy with no nutrition support, or early EN (this time delivered directly into the small bowel via a nasojejunal tube).[54] In the second study the patients on early gastric feeding had problems with tolerance and received significantly less calories and protein than patients on PN.[53] In the third study, tolerance of early nasojejunal feeds was better, such that patients received several calories similar to that received in the PN group.[54] Results were exactly opposite to those reported in the original study by Rapp and colleagues[51] in 1983.[54] In the third study by Charish and colleagues[54] in 1994, pneumonia was significantly more frequent in the PN group (50% vs 18%, $P<.05$) and mortality was significantly higher (23% vs 0%, $P<.05$) when compared with controls receiving early EN. It is ironic that the study by Rapp and colleagues[51] was used to support this meta-analysis by Simpson and Doig,[46] deriving a treatment effect favoring PN that was directly opposite to that of the clinical experience of the original investigators at University of Kentucky.[53,54]

There was another ironic aspect of the meta-analysis by Simpson and Doig[46] and their subjective filter of the literature. Of the 9 studies included in their meta-analysis, none had concealed randomization and only 1 study was blinded.[55] Had they emphasized all the 3 quality components (intent-to-treat analysis, concealed randomization, and appropriate blinding of patients and investigators), they would have been obligated to exclude virtually all of the studies. Instead, they focused only on 1 quality, intent to treat, and as a result, specifically excluded 5 important studies.[53,56–59] As Koretz[60] pointed out in an editorial, there is "no reason to single out one elemental quality as being more important than the others." The 9 studies selected for the meta-analysis by Simpson and Doig[46] still had high risk for bias based on failure to conceal randomization and to blind researchers and patients. Therefore, as Koretz[60] commented, there is "no reason to consider the Simpson-Doig meta-analysis more reliable than any of the others."

The controversy over the preferential use of PN versus EN and the contradictory results of the meta-analysis by Simpson and Doig[46] highlight the difficulties that may arise when subjectivity of a scientific group (such as a guidelines committee) is applied to interpretation of the clinical studies from the literature. Whether the GRADE system[44] succeeds in providing structure for the subjective analysis and whether it improves the transparency of the decisions made by the Guidelines Committee remain to be seen.

SUMMARY

The most important element in the integration of guidelines to clinical practice is transparency, that is, the reader is able to track the recommendation back to the supporting studies. As a large institution, a small group, or a specific individual, it is important to resolve one's own interpretation of each of the controversial issues within a set of guidelines after reviewing the supporting literature. Controversy affords the opportunity for growth and understanding. And yet, the clinician providing nutrition support therapy should understand that with any controversy there may not be a correct answer. The most important step in the conclusion of this process is to determine whether the interpretation of the guidelines and the supportive evidence should alter clinical practice.

REFERENCES

1. McClave SA, Martindale RG, Vanek VW, et al. Guidelines for the provision and assessment of nutrition support therapy in the adult critically ill patient. JPEN J Parenter Eternal Nutr 2009;37(5):277–316.
2. ASPEN Board of Directors and the Clinical Guidelines Task Force. Guidelines for the use of parenteral and enteral nutrition in adult and pediatric patients. JPEN J Parenter Enteral Nutr 2002;26:1SA–138SA.

3. Heyland DK, Dhaliwal R, Drover JW, et al. Canadian clinical practice guidelines for nutrition support in mechanically ventilated, critically ill adult patients. JPEN J Parenter Enteral Nutr 2003;27:355–73.
4. Dellinger RP, Carlet JM, Masur H, et al. Surviving sepsis campaign guidelines for management of severe sepsis and septic shock. Crit Care Med 2004;32(3):858–73.
5. Martindale RG, McClave SA, Vanek VW, et al. Guidelines for the provision and assessment of nutrition support therapy in the adult critically ill patient: Society of Critical Care Medicine (SCCM) and the American Society for Parenteral and Enteral Nutrition (ASPEN): executive summary. Crit Care Med 2009;37(5):1757–61.
6. Choban PS, Dickerson RN. Morbid obesity and nutrition support: is bigger different? Nutr Clin Pract 2005;20:480–7.
7. Bochicchio GV, Joshi M, Bochicchio K, et al. Impact of obesity in the critically ill trauma patient: a prospective study. J Am Coll Surg 2006;203(4):533–8.
8. Bercault N, Boulain T, Kuteifan K, et al. Obesity-related excess mortality rate in an adult intensive care unit: a risk-adjusted matched cohort study. Crit Care Med 2004;32(4):998–1003.
9. Alberda C, Gramlich L, Jones N, et al. The relationship between nutritional intake and clinical outcomes in critically ill patients: results of an international multicenter observational study. Intensive Care Med 2009;35(10):1728–37.
10. Elwyn DH. Nutritional requirements of adult surgical patients. Crit Care Med 1980;8:9–20.
11. Hill GL, Church J. Energy and protein requirements of general surgical patients requiring intravenous nutrition. Br J Surg 1984;71:1–9.
12. Taylor SJ, Fettes SB, Jewkes C, et al. Prospective, randomized, controlled trial to determine the effect of early enhanced enteral nutrition on clinical outcome in mechanically ventilated patients suffering head injury. Crit Care Med 1999;27:2525–31.
13. Pinilla JC, Samphire J, Arnold C, et al. Comparison of gastrointestinal tolerance to two enteral feeding protocols in critically ill patients: a prospective, randomized controlled trial. JPEN J Parenter Enteral Nutr 2001;25(2):81–6.
14. McClave SA, Lukan JK, Stefater JA, et al. Poor validity of residual volumes as a marker for risk of aspiration in critically ill patients. Crit Care Med 2005;33:324–30.
15. Montejo JC, Minambres E, Bordeje L, et al. Gastric residual volume during enteral nutrition in ICU patients: the REGANE study [abstract 0455]. Intensive Care Med 2008. [Epub ahead of print].
16. Powell KS, Marcuard SP, Farrior ES, et al. Aspirating gastric residuals causes occlusion of small-bore feeding tubes. JPEN J Parenter Enteral Nutr 1993;17:243–6.
17. Poulard F, Dimet J, Martin-Levrel A, et al. Impact of not measuring gastric residual volume in mechanically ventilated patients receiving early enteral feeding: a prospective before-afterstudy. JPEN 2010;34(2):125–30.
18. Meissner W, Dohrn B, Reinhart K. Enteral naloxone reduces gastric tube reflux and frequency of pneumonia in critical care patients during opioid analgesia. Crit Care Med 2003;31(3):776–80.
19. Kudsk KA, Croce MA, Fabian TC, et al. Enteral versus parenteral feeding: effects on septic morbidity after blunt and penetrating abdominal trauma. Ann Surg 1992;215:503–13.

20. Heyland DK, Novak F. Immunonutrition in the critically ill patient: more harm than good? JPEN J Parenter Enteral Nutr 2001;25:S51–5.
21. Bower RH, Cerra FB, Bershadsky B, et al. Early enteral administration of a formula (Impact) supplemented with arginine, nucleotides, and fish oil in intensive care unit patients: results of a multicenter, prospective, randomized, clinical trial. Crit Care Med 1995;23(3):436–49.
22. Dent DL, Heyland DK, Levy H, et al. Immunonutrition may increase mortality in critically ill patients with pneumonia: results of a randomized trial. Crit Care Med 2003;30:A17.
23. Bertolini G, Iapichino G, Radrizzani D, et al. Early enteral immunonutrition in patients with severe sepsis: results of an interim analysis of a randomized multi-centre clinical trial. Intensive Care Med 2003;29(5):834–40.
24. Galban C, Montejo JC, Mesejo A, et al. An immune-enhancing enteral diet reduces mortality rate and episodes of bacteremia in septic intensive care unit patients. Crit Care Med 2000;28(3):643–8.
25. Kieft H, Roos A, Bindels A, et al. Clinical outcome of an immune enhancing diet in a heterogenous intensive care population. Intensive Care Med 2005; 31:524–32.
26. Available at: www.criticalcarenutrition.com. Accessed January 2010.
27. Available at: eal@adaevidencelibrary.com. Accessed January 2010.
28. Luiking YC, Poeze M, Preiser J, et al. L-Arginine infusion in severely septic patients does not enhance protein nitrosylation or haemodynamic instability. E-SPEN 2006;1:14–5.
29. Nijveldt RJ, Siroen MP, Teerlink T, et al. Elimination of asymmetric dimethylarginine by the kidney and the liver: a link to the development of multiple organ failure. J Nutr 2004;134:2848S–52.
30. Boger RH. The pharmacodynamics of L-arginine. J Nutr 2007;137:1650S.
31. A prospective, randomized, multi-center trial of initial EDEN-Omega trophic enteral feeding followed by advancement to full calorie enteral feeding vs. early advancement to full calorie enteral feeding in patients with acute lung injury (ALI) or acute respiratory distress syndrome (ARDS) and prospective, randomized, blinded, placebo-controlled multi-center trial of omega-3 fatty acid, gamma-linolenic acid, and anti-oxidant supplementation in management of acute lung injury (ALI) or acute respiratory distress syndrome (ARDS). P.I. Marc Moss. Sponsor: NIH/NHLBI. Available at: www.ardsnet.org/taxonomy/term/135. Accessed October 2009.
32. Herndon DN, Barrow RE, Stein M, et al. Increased mortality with intravenous supplemental feeding in severely burned patients. J Burn Care Rehabil 1989; 10:309–13.
33. Herndon DN, Stein MD, Rutan TC, et al. Failure of TPN supplementation to improve liver function, immunity, and mortality in thermally injured patients. J Trauma 1987;27:195–204.
34. Chiarelli AG, Ferrarello S, Piccioli A, et al. Total enteral nutrition versus mixed enteral and parenteral nutrition in patients in an intensive care unit. Minerva Anestesiol 1996;62:1–7.
35. Bauer P, Charpentier C, Bouchet C, et al. Parenteral with enteral nutrition in the critically ill. Intensive Care Med 2000;26:893–900.
36. Dunham CM, Frankenfield D, Belzberg H, et al. Gut failure-predictor of or contributor to mortality in mechanically ventilated blunt trauma patients? J Trauma 1994; 37(1):30–4.

37. Villet S, Chiolero RL, Bollmann MD, et al. Negative impact of hypocaloric feeding and energy balance on clinical outcome in ICU patients. Clin Nutr 2005;24(4):502–9.
38. Kreymann KG, Berger MM, Deutz NE, et al. ESPEN guidelines on enteral nutrition: intensive care. Clin Nutr 2006;25(2):210–23.
39. Senna MJ, Utter GH, Cuschieri J, et al. Early supplemental parenteral nutrition is associated with increased infectious complications in critically ill trauma patients. J Am Coll Surg 2008;207:459–67.
40. Elke G, Schadler D, Engel C, et al. Current practice in nutrition support and it association with mortality in septic patients—results of a national, prospective, multicenter study. Crit Care Med 2008;36(6):1762–7.
41. Dvir D, Cohen J, Singer P. Computerized energy balance and complications in critically ill patients: an observational study. Clin Nutr 2006;25:37–44.
42. Jain M, Heyland DK, Dhaliwal R, et al. Dissemination of the Canadian clinical practice guidelines for nutrition support: results of a cluster randomized trial. Crit Care Med 2006;34:2362–99.
43. Doig GS, Simpson F, Finfer S, et al. Effect of evidence-based feeding guidelines on mortality of critically ill adults: a cluster randomized controlled trial. JAMA 2008;300(23):2731–41.
44. Available at: www.gradeworkinggroup.org. Accessed April 2010.
45. Bistrian B. Parenteral versus enteral nutrition in the critically ill. JPEN 2010;34(3): 348–9.
46. Simpson F, Doig GS. Parenteral vs. enteral nutrition in the critically ill patient: a meta-analysis of trials using the intention to treat principle. Intensive Care Med 2005;31(1):12–23.
47. Gramlich L, Kichian K, Pinilla J, et al. Does enteral nutrition compared to parenteral nutrition result in better outcomes in critically ill adult patients? A systematic review of the literature. Nutrition 2004;20(10):843–8.
48. Moore FA, Feliciano DV, Andrassy RJ, et al. Early enteral feeding, compared with parenteral, reduces postoperative septic complications: the results of a meta-analysis. Ann Surg 1992;216:172–83.
49. Peter JV, Moran JL, Phillips-Hughes J. A metaanalysis of treatment outcomes of early enteral versus early parenteral nutrition in hospitalized patients. Crit Care Med 2005;33(1):213–20.
50. Heyland DK, Dhaliwal R, Drover JW, et al. Canadian clinical practice guidelines for nutrition support in mechanically ventilated critically ill adult patients. JPEN 2003;27:355–73.
51. Rapp RP, Young DB, Twyman D. The favorable effect of early parenteral feeding on survival in head-injured patients. J Neurosurg 1983;58:906–12.
52. Woodcock NP, Zeigler D, Palmer MD, et al. Enteral versus parenteral nutrition: a pragmatic study. Nutrition 2001;17:1–12.
53. Young B, Ott L, Haack D. Effect of total parenteral nutrition upon intracranial pressure in severe head injury. J Neurosurg 1987;67:76–80.
54. Charash WE, Kearney PA, Annus KA, et al. Early enteral feeding is associated with an attenuation of the acute phase/cytokine response and improved outcome following multiple trauma. J Trauma 1994;37:1015.
55. Rayes R, Hansen S, Seehofer D, et al. Early enteral supply of fiber and Lactobacilli versus conventional nutrition: a controlled trial in patients with major abdominal surgery. Nutrition 2002;18:609–15.
56. Moore FA, Moore EE, Jones TN, et al. TEN versus TPN following major abdominal trauma—reduced septic morbidity. J Trauma 1989;29(7):916–23.

57. Kalfarentzos F, Kehagias J, Mead N, et al. Enteral nutrition is superior to parenteral nutrition in severe acute pancreatitis: results of a randomized prospective trial. Br J Surg 1997;84:1665–9.
58. Cerra FB, McPherson JP, Konstantinides FN, et al. Enteral nutrition does not prevent multiple organ failure syndrome (MOFS) after sepsis. Surgery 1988; 104:727–33.
59. Borzotta AP, Pennings J, Papasadero B, et al. Enteral versus parenteral nutrition after severe closed head injury. J Trauma 1994;37(3):459–68.
60. Koretz RL. Carts, horses, and evidence. JPEN J Parenter Eternal Nutr 2008;32(4): 482–5.

Parenteral Nutrition in Critical Illness: Can it Safely Improve Outcomes?

Ronan Thibault, MD, PhD[a,b], Claude Pichard, MD, PhD[a,*]

KEYWORDS

• Enteral nutrition • Supplemental parenteral nutrition
• Undernutrition • Protein–energy deficit • Intensive care unit

Total parenteral nutrition (TPN) was developed at the end of the 1950s,[1] and its use increased rapidly in the 1960s to 1970s. TPN was then widely implemented in intensive care units (ICU) and considered as the first-line nutrition support. During this time, TPN was not administered according to the all-in-one principle, so that macronutrients (ie, glucose, lipids, amino acids) were administered separately and with inconsistent flow rates. Moreover, the extensive and systematic use of TPN in ICUs was based on the paradigm that the more calories a patients received the better their outcome. Unfortunately, as a result, TPN administration was associated with overfeeding and related metabolic disorders, leading to increased morbidity and mortality. The technique of enteral nutrition (EN), which is believed to be more physiologic, was developed and since the 1980s, progressively replaced TPN as the gold standard nutritional therapy in patients in the ICU. As a result, early EN is now recommended by current guidelines as the first indicated feeding route in these patients.[2–4] However, recent literature indicates that EN alone is often unable to fully meet the nutritional needs,[5–8] thus inducing a cumulated protein–energy deficit that is associated with a worse clinical outcome.[9–12] The medical environment and patients are changing: medical technology has improved (eg, better mechanical ventilation, infection control, and hemodynamic management), more patients are elderly, obesity is more widespread, the prevalence of chronic diseases has increased (ie, cancer, degenerative neurologic diseases, organ insufficiency), and more people are living a sedentary lifestyle. Patients with preexisting undernutrition or lean tissue depletion (eg, sarcopenic

This work was supported by grants from the Société Nationale Française de Gastroentérologie (SNFGE) and the public Nutrition 2000 Plus foundation.

a Nutrition Unit, Geneva University Hospital, Rue Gabrielle-Perret-Gentil, 4, 1211 Geneva 14, Switzerland
b Department of Gastroenterology and Nutrition Support, UMR 1280 PhAN, CRNH Nantes, IMAD, CHU Nantes, 1 place A. Ricordeau, 44093 Nantes Cedex 01, Nantes, France
* Corresponding author.
E-mail address: claude.pichard@unige.ch

obesity) are becoming prevalent. Because these conditions are incompatible with stress-induced catabolism and rapid healing and recovery, the prevention of their onset or worsening is vital. Therefore, currently, after patients undergo two consecutive periods of TPN alone, then EN alone, the nutritional support needs to be reconsidered as a way of optimizing lean body mass and protein–energy balance during the first week after ICU admission. This concept is based on the assertion that limiting the energy debt should improve the clinical outcome and shorten the recovery period.

After an overview of the past and present context of the use of nutrition support in ICU, this article shows that combining EN with parenteral nutrition (PN) may represent the best option for preventing protein–energy deficit in ICU patients, and supports the logical hypothesis that, in the near future, the combination of PN and EN could improve the clinical outcome of ICU patients if EN alone is not feasible or suboptimal.

THE BEGINNINGS OF PARENTERAL IN THE INTENSIVE CARE UNIT: "PARENTERAL NUTRITION IS A POISON THERAPY"

Before the 1980s, the gold standard of nutritional management in the ICU was TPN. Patients received high-caloric delivery based on the belief that the higher calories patients received the better their outcome. Also, the excess administration of calories, particularly from carbohydrates and fats, the so-called hyperalimentation or overfeeding, was promoted as a means to enhance recovery from disease.[13] This period of systematic and widespread use of TPN corresponds with the beginning of modern intensive care medicine. In that context, most critically ill patients died within the first days of ICU stay from shock, multiple organ failure, or acute respiratory distress syndrome. The impact of nutritional support was therefore minor. When improvements in intensive care medicine began to prevent critically ill patients from experiencing early death, severe metabolic and infectious complications began to be observed during the early postinjury phase, related to TPN.[13–15] The high rate of infectious complications was often related to hyperglycemia.[13–15] These observations led Marik and Pinsky[15] to call TPN a "poison therapy."

In the past 20 years, studies extensively showed that TPN could induce metabolic disorders, such as hyperglycemia, hypertriglyceridemia and liver steatosis, endocrine dysfunction, impairment of immunity, infections; and increased mortality.[13–15] Intestinal mucosal atrophy, leading to bacterial translocation from the gut to the bloodstream, was proposed as a theoretical complication of PN and was implicated in the increased incidence of infection and sepsis seen with PN.[13] However, human studies have found that PN given in the setting of complete bowel rest did not result in intestinal atrophy, even after a month of no enteral intake.[13] Furthermore, evidence does not show that the risk for bacterial translocation is increased by TPN.[13,16]

Thus, TPN has been associated with several theoretical and actual complications, leading to restriction of its use and the development of EN. However, commercially available PN solutions have evolved considerably during the past 2 decades. As a result, all-in-one solutions are now widely implemented in the ICU. This method of administration allows a lower and constant load of glucose and lipid substrates to be obtained, reducing the risk for hyperglycemia, hypertriglyceridemia, and liver fat overload. The composition of lipids emulsions has also evolved. The increased use of the mix of long- and medium-chain triglycerides and of olive oil–enriched lipid emulsions has likely reduced the risk for TPN-related metabolic and liver complications. Therefore, studies performed before 1990 likely do not reflect current clinical practice.

THE RECENT PAST OF NUTRITION SUPPORT IN THE INTENSIVE CARE UNIT: "ENTERAL NUTRITION IS SAFER AND MORE PHYSIOLOGIC"

From a physiologic point of view, in critically ill patients with an intact and functional gastrointestinal tract, enteral feeding through nasogastric tube, gastrostomy, or jejunostomy is recommended as first-line nutritional support when oral feeding is impossible.[2–4] EN is believed to offer several advantages over the parenteral route for the delivery of nutrition. EN is believed to be more physiologic, may help restore or maintain intestinal trophicity, may improve immune and gut-barrier function, and has been associated with a reduced risk for infectious complications in ICU patients compared with PN.[3,17–19] EN offers metabolic benefits, such as better regulation of insulin secretion, glycemia, and lipid clearance, which in turn reduce the risk for hepatic dysfunction and overfeeding-related complications. EN also reduces the risk for refeeding syndrome.

Finally, EN has also been associated with cost savings in the ICU.[20,21] For example, an annual net profit of $357,000 was estimated to result from optimizing the use of EN in lieu of PN in the ICU of a single hospital in Sweden.[21] However, the costs of nutritional therapy have to be counterbalanced with the costs of nutritional support–related complications or side effects. For example, the prevalence of diarrhea may vary from 2% to 95% in ICU patients, and the administration of EN is often complicated with diarrhea.[22] It is well-known that diarrhea is associated with increased costs of materials (antibiotics, bedclothes, gloves, rectal tubes, and other disposable items), nursing time (changes of bedclothes and disposable diapers, or rectal tubes), and medical time (prescriptions and investigations related to diarrhea). Thus, the cost of EN-related diarrhea could equal or exceed the overall cost of TPN or combined EN and PN in ICU. A prospective study protocol is currently verifying this hypothesis.

The timing of EN initiation seems to be a clinically important factor; specifically, early initiation of EN in ICU patients has been associated with improved outcomes. In a retrospective analysis of more than 4000 nonsurgical, mechanically ventilated, critically ill patients, ICU mortality, hospital mortality, and length of ICU stay were significantly reduced in patients who received EN within 48 hours of mechanical ventilation initiation versus those who did not.[23] Early EN also has been shown to decrease the rate of infectious complications, total length of hospital stay, and overall costs of patient management in postsurgical patients.[24,25] Several studies or meta-analyses have shown consistent benefit of early EN in decreasing infectious complications, overall hospital and ICU lengths of stay, costs, and mortality.[7,8,17,24,26,27] A retrospective cohort study conducted in a medical ICU found greater mortality with delayed EN than with early EN.[23]

Implementation of early EN has therefore become standard practice in ICU patients and is advocated in several clinical guidelines.[2–4] However, the clinical benefit of EN could be limited in some subgroups of patients. For instance, mortality and infection rates were shown to be higher in undernourished patients treated with EN than in those treated with PN.[18] This finding deserves to be evaluated in patients with sarcopenia.

THE PRESENT: WHY DOES PARENTERAL NUTRITION NEED TO BE RECONSIDERED IN THE MANAGEMENT OF INTENSIVE CARE UNIT PATIENTS?
Enteral Nutrition is Associated with a Protein–energy Deficit

Since the wide implementation of EN alone as the preferred nutritional support in ICUs, numerous studies have shown that EN was insufficient to cover protein and energy requirements (**Fig. 1**).[5–8] In daily practice, achieving targeted nutritional goals with EN

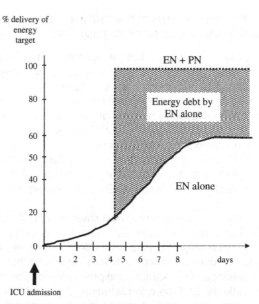

Fig. 1. The combination of enteral and parenteral nutrition (EN + PN) in ICU patients. Use of enteral nutrition alone (*solid line*) is frequently associated with an energy debt that cannot be compensated for later. The association of EN with supplemental PN (*dotted line*) allows early and optimal (ie, 100%) coverage of the energy target. Overfeeding must be avoided because it is related to an increased risk for hyperglycemia, infections, and death.

is often difficult. Optimal implementation of EN in the ICU remains a challenge even when a well-trained and experienced nutrition team is available.[5] EN is frequently interrupted in ICU patients for multiple and recurrent events, such as radiologic or endoscopic investigations, surgery, and technical problems with pumps or feeding tubes.[7] Also, initiation of EN is often delayed because of concerns about gastrointestinal intolerance (eg, vomiting, diarrhea, abdominal distention) and dysmotility (gastroparesis, ileus), which occurs in as many as 46% of patients receiving nutrients by this route.[28]

Insufficient EN delivery is also seen because of inaccurate medical prescriptions or inadequate routine nursing procedures, such as repeated gastric residues measurements. Analyses conducted in ICUs in the United States[29] and Canada[30] found that of the total calories prescribed, only 52% and 56%, respectively, were actually delivered through the enteral route to the patients in these units. In United States centers, compliance with a standardized enteral feeding protocol only improved the delivery of calories to 68% of the target amount.[29] In 494 ICU patients, Genton and colleagues[5] showed that on day 5, fewer than 30% received 90% or more of the prescribed calories, and their protein delivery reached only approximately 70% of requirements; clearly an underfeeding of the patients.

The implementation of feeding protocols has been proposed as a strategy to optimize nutritional support.[31] The Critical-Care Enteral and Parenteral Therapy (ACCEPT) study, a Canadian study conducted in 14 hospitals,[32] showed that survival from intensive care improved when evidence-based guidelines for nutrition were followed and larger amounts of nutrition were delivered more consistently. However, others showed that the implementation of nutritional support protocols was disappointing, because only approximately 60%[30] of ICU patients included in the protocols could achieve their energy targets.

The concept of early EN, based on an excellent physiologic approach, is often associated with failure to achieve energy targets. Therefore, during the early phase after ICU admission, a negative protein–energy balance is frequently observed and cannot be compensated for later.[9,10]

Influence of Undernutrition and Negative Energy Balance on Clinical Outcome

The combination of stress-induced catabolism and insufficient coverage of energy target by EN alone is associated with negative energy balance, which leads to lean body mass loss and undernutrition (**Fig. 2**).[33] Catabolism of lean body mass has been repeatedly associated with a worsening of the clinical outcome (ie, increased rate of infections and multiple organ failure), delayed wound healing, prolonged

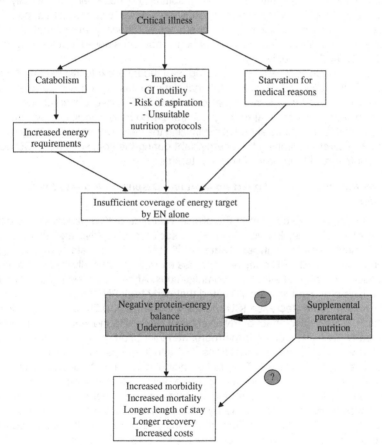

Fig. 2. Impact of the use of enteral nutrition (EN) alone during critical illness. Critical illness is associated with a catabolism of lean body mass, and starvation for medical reasons is regularly ordered. EN is difficult to optimize in the context of gastrointestinal (GI) intolerance, risk for aspiration, and unsuitable nursing or medical nutrition protocols. Thus, the use of EN is associated with an insufficient coverage of the energy target. As a consequence, the protein–energy deficit leads to the onset of undernutrition or the impairment of preexisting undernutrition, which are associated with a worse clinical outcome. Through reducing the protein–energy deficit, supplemental parenteral nutrition could improve the clinical outcome.

mechanical ventilation, increased length of hospital stay and recovery, increased mortality,[34-37] and, ultimately, increased global health care costs.[36,38] The risk for severe undernutrition during the ICU stay is further increased because patients are frequently undernourished before their admission into the ICU; up to 50% of patients admitted to European hospitals have various degrees of undernutrition.[35,36,39]

The inability to deliver adequate energy intake, resulting in a negative protein–energy balance, has been associated with increased morbidity and mortality in ICU patients.[6,9,10,23,26,36] In medical and surgical ICU patients, hypocaloric feeding is associated with increased risk for complications, such as infection rate,[9-11] impaired wound healing,[10] adult respiratory distress syndrome, renal failure, need for surgery, and pressure sores.[10] The increased rate of complications related to undernutrition and energy deficit leads to an increase in hospital length of stay and costs.[35,36,38,39] In a Brazilian study of 709 patients from 25 hospitals, the mean per-patient daily health care costs were 61% higher for malnourished versus well-nourished patients.[36] In Europe, the mean overall hospital costs for nutritionally at-risk patients were more than double those incurred by patients not considered nutritionally at-risk (4891 € vs 2204 €, respectively).[38]

Despite several corrective measures proposed recently, exclusive use of EN in ICU patients remains associated with nutritional deficiencies, which are correlated with impaired short- and long-term clinical outcomes.[32,34] These observations support the need for early and optimal (during the first 24 hours of the ICU stay) nutritional management of ICU patients aimed at minimizing the negative protein–energy balance (see **Fig. 2**). Therefore, limiting the energy debt during the first week after ICU admission is hypothesized to improve clinical outcome.

Parenteral Nutrition Has No Impact on Mortality Despite an Increased Rate of Infections

Numerous studies have compared the clinical outcome of ICU patients according to the route of feeding (ie, EN vs PN or EN associated with PN), and this has been included in several meta-analyses (**Table 1**).[3,18,20,40-42] These meta-analyses suggest that, compared with EN, PN does not increase mortality in critically ill patients despite an increased incidence of infectious complications. After evaluating 465 publications, a meta-analysis of eight studies indicated that early total PN compared with delayed EN (>24 hours) could decrease ICU mortality (odds ratio, 0.29; 95% CI, 0.12–0.70; $P = .006$).[42] This positive effect of PN on survival was not found when comparing early PN with early EN (<24 hours). Furthermore, administration of early PN has also been associated with increased complications,[15,45] although this may be related to overfeeding rather than to PN itself. The studies included in the meta-analysis raise methodological issues: patient populations were very heterogeneous, including two studying only burn patients, and all studies were performed before 1998, when hyperglycemia was frequent because the benefits of glycemic control had not yet been shown.[13,44] Thus, the results of this meta-analysis are not sufficient to conclude absence of clinical benefit associated with EN/PN versus EN alone.

Other studies show that PN is associated with an increased risk for infections.[3,20,42,45] Recent multicenter studies of ICU patients indicate that the use of PN or its duration of use is associated with an increased risk for Candida colonization or candidemia.[46,47] However, other independent risk factors of Candida infections have been identified, including sepsis, multifocal colonization, and surgery.[47] An Italian multicentric randomized study conducted in 33 general ICUs found that the 28-day mortality did not differ between patients receiving early enteral immunonutrition or PN (15.6% vs 15.1%; P value not significant).[48] However, in the subgroup of

Table 1
Simplified results of the meta-analyses comparing enteral nutrition and parenteral nutrition[a] in patients in the intensive care unit

References	Number of Studies Included (n)	Mortality Risk Associated with EN vs PN	Infections Risk Associated with EN vs PN
Braunschweig et al[18]	20	1.14 [0.69–1.88]	0.77 [0.65–0.91]*
	7 (undernourished patients)	3.0 [1.09–8.56]*	1.17 [0.88–1.56]
Heyland et al[3]	12	1.08 [0.70–1.65]	0.61 [0.44–0.84]**
Dhaliwal et al[40]	5 (#EN vs EN + PN)	1.27 [0.82–1.94]	1.14 [0.66–1.96]
Gramlich et al[20]	13	1.08 [0.70–1.65]	0.64 [0.47–0.87]*
Peter et al[41]	24	0.01 [−0.01–0.02]†	0.08 [0.04–0.12]†**
Simpson and Doig[42]	11	0.51 [0.27–0.97]*	1.66 [1.09–2.51]*

Favours PN Favours EN   Favours PN Favours EN

No effect of parenteral nutrition on mortality is shown. Odds ratio [95% confidence interval] are indicated in the boxes, except for †risk difference [95% confidence interval].

Abbreviations: EN, enteral nutrition; PN, parenteral nutrition.
* $P < .05$; ** $P < .01$.
[a] Except #EN.

Data from Singer P, Berger MM, van den Berghe G, et al. ESPEN Guidelines on parenteral nutrition: intensive care. Clin Nutr 2009;28:387–400; and Heidegger CP, Darmon P, Pichard C. Enteral vs. parenteral nutrition for the critically ill patient: a combined support should be preferred. Curr Opin Crit Care 2007;14:408–14.

patients without septic shock (n = 142), the administration of PN was associated with more episodes of severe sepsis or septic shock (13.1% vs 4.9%; P = .02). In another study performed in 415 patients with severe sepsis or septic shock from 454 ICUs, the use of PN was independently associated with an increased risk for death after adjustment for patient morbidity.[49] In trauma patients with good EN tolerance, early PN was associated with an increased infectious morbidity.[48] However, a randomized controlled study performed in patients with brain trauma found no differences in duration of mechanical ventilation, survival, or long-term sequelae between patients treated with EN and those treated with PN.[19]

In summary, PN does not affect mortality contrary to former beliefs, except in patients with severe septic shock. Overall, PN alone is associated with an increased risk for infectious complications, which is further increased by the duration of PN and presence of other factors, such as sepsis, recent surgery, and multifocal colonization. Therefore, in selected patients, it may be hypothesized that modern all-in-one PN can be administered successfully and safely if by a trained team,[5,13,16] energy delivery is adapted to the energy target (ie, overfeeding is avoided), glycemic control is observed,[50,51] and PN is limited to only when absolutely needed.[44] These observations prompt reconsideration of PN use when EN is insufficient to meet the energy target (see **Fig. 1**), as indicated by recent guidelines (**Table 2**).

Influence of the Timing of Nutritional Support on Clinical Outcome

The timing nutritional support initiation and amounts of energy delivered perhaps may be more important then the route of feeding (ie, EN, PN). One study involving 1209 ICU patients showed that early EN or PN that achieved the energy target in the 3 first days of ICU stay was associated with decreased morbidity and mortality.[52] Another study of 150 patients receiving mechanical ventilation showed that, although initiated within the first 24 hours, EN delivering less than 28% of the estimated caloric and protein requirements increased infection rate and lengthened hospital stay compared with a progressive increase in calorie delivery over 5 days.[31] Another investigation showed a reduction in the duration of mechanical ventilation associated with improved nutritional support.[12]

THE FUTURE: OPTIMIZATION OF NUTRITION SUPPORT BY SUPPLEMENTAL PARENTERAL NUTRITION TOGETHER WITH ENTERAL NUTRITION
Impact of Supplemental Parenteral Nutrition on Achieving Energy Target and Adequate Nutritional Status

Box 1 summarizes the previously reported and presumed advantages of the combination of PN and EN in ICU patients. Studies have shown that PN could allow a higher proportion of the energy target to be achieved than EN alone.[7,53] The implementation of combination EN + PN should be able to match energy requirements with delivery (see **Fig. 1**).

Recently, the authors published an abstract[54] reporting the preliminary results of a prospective, controlled, randomized study investigating whether the delivery of 100% of the energy target in ICU patients from day 4 by EN + supplemental parenteral nutrition (SPN) could optimize clinical outcome (www.clinicaltrials.gov, study protocol #NCT00802503). They showed that the mean energy delivery from day 4 to 8 was significantly higher with EN + SPN than with EN alone (98.0 ± 19.0 vs 80.0 ± 31.7; P<.001).[54] Another study confirms that combined nutritional support with EN + SPN increases calorie delivery compared with EN alone (2160 vs 1365 kcal/d; P<.0001).[9] These findings suggest that the combination of EN + PN could also achieve protein needs sooner during critical illness. In a study of 49 undernourished ICU patients

Table 2
Summary of current guidelines concerning the timing of the initiation of PN and the indications of supplemental PN together with EN in critically ill patients[a]

ESPEN[2,43]	ASPEN[4]	Canadian Guidelines[3]
1. PN should be avoided in patients who tolerate EN and are meeting their energy target (A).	1. Nutrition support therapy in the form of EN should be initiated in critically ill patients unable to maintain volitional intake (C).	1. For critically ill patients starting on EN, recommendation is that PN not be started at the same time (B).
2. All patients who are not expected to be on normal nutrition within 3 days should receive PN within 24–48 h if EN is contraindicated or they cannot tolerate EN (C).	2. If early EN is not feasible or available over the first 7 days after admission to the ICU, no nutrition support therapy should be provided in non-undernourished patients (C). In previously undernourished patients, PN should be initiated as soon as possible after admission and adequate resuscitation (C).	2. and 3. In patients not tolerating adequate EN, data are insufficient to recommend when PN should be initiated (B).
3. All patients receiving less than their targeted enteral feeding after 2 days should be considered for supplemental PN (B).	3. Initiating supplemental PN before this 7- to 10-day period in patients already on EN does not improve outcome and may be detrimental (C).	

Abbreviations: ASPEN, American Society for Parenteral and Enteral Nutrition; EN, enteral nutrition; ESPEN, European Society for Clinical Nutrition and Metabolism; ICU, intensive care unit; PN, parenteral nutrition.
[a] The level of recommendations according to the evidence-based medicine classification is indicated in parentheses.

Box 1
Advantages of the combination of enteral nutrition and parenteral nutrition for the management of critically ill patients

Proven advantages

Increased coverage of energy target

Improved protein–energy balance

Presumed advantages

Maintenance of intestinal trophicity

Maintenance of immune and gut-barrier function

Reduced risk for overnutrition and its metabolic complications (hyperglycemia, insulinoresistance, hypertriglyceridemia, liver steatosis)

Reduced risk for infections

Better gastrointestinal tolerance: reduced risk for vomiting, gastroesophageal reflux, diarrhea

Reduced risk for aspiration and pneumonia

---

receiving mechanical ventilation, serum transthyretin and the Maastricht index (an assessment tool of nutritional status that incorporates serum transthyretin and albumin, lymphocyte count, and percentage of ideal weight) significantly increased after 2 weeks of combined nutrition support, whereas no improvement was observed in patients treated with EN or PN alone.[55] This effect could be related to the increase in energy delivery.[56]

These observations support the concept that SPN could optimize nutritional therapy when EN does not allow achieving the energy target. In addition, the authors believe that the early use of combined EN + SPN could have a positive impact on protein–energy balance and clinical outcome (see **Fig. 1**). Three randomized controlled trials are underway to confirm whether combining insufficient EN with PN has beneficial effects on clinical outcome and economic aspects.

Current and Putative Indications of Supplemental Parenteral Nutrition in the Intensive Care Unit

The European Society for Clinical Nutrition and Metabolism (ESPEN) guidelines on EN in the ICU recommend that, in the acute phase of critical illness, patients should receive a maximum of 20 to 25 kcal/kg per day, increasing to 25 to 30 kcal/kg per day during recovery.[2] Severely malnourished patients should receive a maximum of 25 to 30 kcal/kg per day from the time that feeding is initiated.[2] If these nutritional goals cannot be achieved using EN alone, the American and European guidelines[4,43] recommend that supplemental PN be initiated. As shown in **Table 2**, the optimal time to initiate supplemental PN is still debated. As early PN may be superior to delayed EN,[42] ESPEN recommends that PN be administered to all ICU patients in whom EN cannot be initiated within 24 hours of ICU admission or injury.[43] A similar recommendation is made by the American Society for Parenteral and Enteral Nutrition (ASPEN), which advises the use of PN as soon as possible only for undernourished patients in whom EN is not feasible.[4] For patients with no evidence of protein-calorie malnutrition, PN should be initiated after the first 7 days of hospitalization.[4] The authors proposed initiating PN to achieve 100% of energy and protein targets by day 4 when EN fails to meet 60% of the patient's nutritional needs within 3 days.[44] A sequential approach should be considered and PN gradually weaned as EN reaches the energy target, to avoid overfeeding and infectious complications of PN.

Given the association between hyperglycemia and increased morbidity and mortality in critically ill patients, glycemic control should be ensured during combined EN and PN, with the goal of obtaining a glycemia less than 10 mmol/L.[50] Hypoglycemia must be avoided.[51] Reaching an adequacy between nutritional needs and prescription is mandatory to avoid protein–energy deficit, overfeeding, and hyperglycemia, and the onset of their related complications.

SUMMARY

TPN, administered with separated macronutrients and inconsistent flow rates, was first considered the gold standard of nutrition therapy in ICU, but was associated with overnutrition and its metabolic complications. This resulted in increased mortality and infectious morbidity. Thus, EN alone, believed to be more physiologic, has progressively replaced PN as the gold standard of nutritional care in ICU. However, EN alone is frequently associated with insufficient coverage of energy requirements and subsequent protein–energy deficit, which is correlated with a worsened clinical outcome. Recent evidence suggests that all-in-one PN has no significant negative effect on mortality and infectious morbidity in ICU patients. After these two distinct periods of prioritizing use of PN followed by EN, the combination of both techniques may be a better strategy to improve calorie delivery, reduce protein–energy deficit, and perhaps, improve clinical outcome and global health care costs. Consideration of this combination is vital for the future, because the combination of aging, sarcopenic obesity, chronic diseases, and preexisting undernutrition increases vulnerability to stress-related catabolism in ICU patients. Clinical studies are warranted to confirm that the combination of PN and EN can reduce undernutrition-related morbidity and mortality, and improve recovery after the ICU stay.

ACKNOWLEDGMENTS

R. Thibault is supported by research grants from the Société Nationale Française de Gastroentérologie (SNFGE) and the public Nutrition 2000 Plus foundation.

REFERENCES

1. Wretlind A. The possibilities of providing adequate parenteral nutrition. Nord Med 1955;53(26):1013–9.
2. Kreymann KG, Berger MM, Deutz NE, et al. ESPEN guidelines on enteral nutrition: intensive care. Clin Nutr 2006;25:210–23.
3. Heyland DK, Dhaliwal R, Drover JW, et al. Canadian Critical Care Clinical Practice Guidelines Committee. Canadian clinical practice guidelines for nutrition support in mechanically ventilated, critically ill adult patients. J Parenter Enteral Nutr 2003; 27:355–73.
4. Martindale R, McClave S, Vanek V, et al. Guidelines for the provision and assessment of nutrition support therapy in the adult critically ill patient: Society of Critical Care Medicine and American Society for Parenteral and Enteral Nutrition: executive summary. Crit Care Med 2009;37:1757–61.
5. Genton L, Dupertuis YM, Romand JA, et al. Higher calorie prescription improves nutrient delivery during the first 5 days of enteral nutrition. Clin Nutr 2004;23: 307–15.

6. Kyle UG, Genton L, Heidegger CP, et al. Hospitalized mechanically ventilated patients are at higher risk of enteral underfeeding than nonventilated patients. Clin Nutr 2006;25:727–35.

7. De Jonghe B, Appere-De-Vechi C, Fournier M, et al. A prospective survey of nutritional support practices in intensive care unit patients: what is prescribed? What is delivered? Crit Care Med 2001;29:8–12.

8. Mackenzie SL, Zygun DA, Whitmore BL, et al. Implementation of a nutrition support protocol increases the proportion of mechanically ventilated patients reaching enteral nutrition targets in the adult intensive care unit. J Parenter Enteral Nutr 2005;29:74–80.

9. Villet S, Chiolero RL, Bollmann MD, et al. Negative impact of hypocaloric feeding and energy balance on clinical outcome in ICU patients. Clin Nutr 2005;24:502–9.

10. Dvir D, Cohen J, Singer P. Computerized energy balance and complications in critically ill patients: an observational study. Clin Nutr 2006;25:37–44.

11. Rubinson L, Diette GB, Song X, et al. Low caloric intake is associated with noso-comial bloodstream infections in patients in the medical intensive care unit. Crit Care Med 2004;32:350–7.

12. Barr J, Hecht M, Flavin KE, et al. Outcomes in critically ill patients before and after the implementation of an evidence-based nutritional management protocol. Chest 2004;125:1446–57.

13. Jeejeebhoy KN. Total parenteral nutrition: potion or poison? Am J Clin Nutr 2001; 74:160–3.

14. Ziegler TR. Parenteral nutrition in the critically ill patient. N Engl J Med 2009;361: 1088–97.

15. Marik PE, Pinsky M. Death by parenteral nutrition. Intensive Care Med 2003;29: 867–9.

16. Nardo P, Dupertuis YM, Jetzer J, et al. Clinical relevance of parenteral nutrition prescription and administration in 200 hospitalized patients: a quality control study. Clin Nutr 2008;27:858–64.

17. Dissanaike S, Pham T, Shalhub S, et al. Effect of immediate enteral feeding on trauma patients with an open abdomen: protection from nosocomial infections. J Am Coll Surg 2008;207:690–7.

18. Braunschweig CL, Levy P, Sheean PM, et al. Enteral compared with parenteral nutrition: a meta-analysis. Am J Clin Nutr 2001;74:534–42.

19. Koretz RL, Avenell A, Lipman TO, et al. Does enteral nutrition affect clinical outcome? A systematic review of the randomized trials. Am J Gastroenterol 2007;102:412–29.

20. Gramlich L, Kichian K, Pinilla J, et al. Does enteral nutrition compared to paren-teral nutrition result in better outcomes in critically ill adult patients? A systematic review of the literature. Nutrition 2004;20:843–8.

21. Johansson C, Backman L, Jakobsson J. Is enteral nutrition optimally used in hospitalized patients? A study of the practice of nutrition in a Swedish hospital. Clin Nutr 1996;15:171–4.

22. Wiesen P, van Gossum A, Preiser JC. Diarrhoea in the critically ill. Curr Opin Crit Care 2006;12:149–54.

23. Artinian V, Krayem H, DiGiovine B. Effects of early enteral feeding on the outcome of critically ill mechanically ventilated medical patients. Chest 2006; 129:960–7.

24. Neumayer LA, Smout RJ, Horn HG, et al. Early and sufficient feeding reduces length of stay and charges in surgical patients. J Surg Res 2001; 95:73–7.

25. Hedberg AM, Lairson DR, Aday LA, et al. Economic implications of an early post-operative enteral feeding protocol. J Am Diet Assoc 1999;99:802–7.
26. Marik PE, Zaloga GP. Early enteral nutrition in acutely ill patients: a systematic review. Crit Care Med 2001;29:2264–70.
27. Doig GS, Heighes PT, Simpson F, et al. Early enteral nutrition, provided within 24 h of injury or intensive care unit admission, significantly reduces mortality in critically ill patients: a meta-analysis of randomised controlled trials. Intensive Care Med 2009;35(12):2018–27.
28. Mentec H, Dupont H, Bocchetti M, et al. Upper digestive intolerance during enteral nutrition in critically ill patients: frequency, risk factors, and complications. Crit Care Med 2001;29:1955–61.
29. Spain DA, McClave SA, Sexton LK, et al. Infusion protocol improves delivery of enteral tube feeding in the critical care unit. JPEN J Parenter Enteral Nutr 1999; 23:288–92.
30. Sigalet DL, Mackenzie SL, Hameed SM. Enteral nutrition and mucosal immunity: implications for feeding strategies in surgery and trauma. Can J Surg 2004;47: 109–16.
31. Ibrahim EH, Mehringer L, Prentice D, et al. Early versus late enteral feeding of mechanically ventilated patients: results of a clinical trial. J Parenter Enteral Nutr 2002;26:174–81.
32. Martin CM, Doig GS, Heyland DK, et al. Southwestern Ontario Critical Care Research Network. Multicentre, cluster-randomized clinical trial of algorithms for Critical-Care Enteral and Parenteral Therapy (ACCEPT). Can Med Assoc J 2004;170:197–204.
33. Reid CL, Campbell IT, Little RA. Muscle wasting and energy balance in critical illness. Clin Nutr 2004;23:273–80.
34. Kyle UG, Schneider SM, Pirlich M, et al. Does nutritional risk, as assessed by Nutritional Risk Index, increase during hospital stay? A multinational population-based study. Clin Nutr 2005;24:516–24.
35. Pichard C, Kyle UG, Morabia A, et al. Nutritional assessment: lean body mass depletion at hospital admission is associated with increased length of stay. Am J Clin Nutr 2004;79:613–8.
36. Correia MITD, Waitzberg DL. The impact of malnutrition on morbidity, mortality, length of hospital stay and costs evaluated through a multivariate model analysis. Clin Nutr 2003;22:235–9.
37. Ray DE, Matchett SC, Baker K, et al. The effect of body mass index on patient outcomes in a medical ICU. Chest 2005;127:2125–31.
38. Amaral TF, Matos LC, Tavares MM, et al. The economic impact of disease-related malnutrition at hospital admission. Clin Nutr 2007;26:778–84.
39. Pirlich M, Schütz T, Norman K, et al. The German hospital malnutrition study. Clin Nutr 2006;25:563–72.
40. Dhaliwal R, Jurewitsch B, Harrietha D, et al. Combination enteral and parenteral nutrition in critically ill patients: harmful or beneficial? A systematic review of the evidence. Intensive Care Med 2004;30:1666–71.
41. Peter JV, Moran JL, Phillips-Hughes J. A meta-analysis of treatment outcomes of early enteral versus early parenteral nutrition in hospitalized patients. Crit Care Med 2005;33:213–20.
42. Simpson F, Doig GS. Parenteral vs. enteral nutrition in the critically ill patient: a meta-analysis of trials using the intention to treat principle. Intensive Care Med 2005;31:12–23.
43. Singer P, Berger MM, van den Berghe G, et al. ESPEN Guidelines on parenteral nutrition: intensive care. Clin Nutr 2009;28:387–400.

44. Heidegger CP, Darmon P, Pichard C. Enteral vs. parenteral nutrition for the critically ill patient: a combined support should be preferred. Curr Opin Crit Care 2007;14:408–14.
45. Sena MJ, Utter GH, Cuschieri J, et al. Early supplemental parenteral nutrition is associated with increased infectious complications in critically ill trauma patients. J Am Coll Surg 2008;207:459–67.
46. Chow JK, Golan Y, Ruthazer R, et al. Risk factors for albicans and non-albicans candidemia in the intensive care unit. Crit Care Med 2008;36:1993–8.
47. León C, Alvarez-Lerma F, Ruiz-Santana S, et al. EPCAN Study Group. Fungal colonization and/or infection in non-neutropenic critically ill patients: results of the EPCAN observational study. Eur J Clin Microbiol Infect Dis 2009;28:233–42.
48. Radrizzani D, Bertolini G, Facchini R, et al. Early enteral immunonutrition vs. parenteral nutrition in critically ill patients without severe sepsis: a randomized clinical trial. Intensive Care Med 2006;32:1191–8.
49. Elke G, Schädler D, Engel C, et al. German Competence Network Sepsis (SepNet). Current practice in nutritional support and its association with mortality in septic patients-results from a national, prospective, multicenter study. Crit Care Med 2008;36:1762–7.
50. NICE-SUGAR Study Investigators, Finfer S, Chittock DR, Su SY, et al. Intensive versus conventional glucose control in critically ill patients. N Engl J Med 2009; 360:1283–97.
51. Van den Berghe G, Wilmer A, Hermans G, et al. Intensive insulin therapy in the medical ICU. N Engl J Med 2006;354:449–61.
52. Pichard C, Kreymann GK, Weimann A, et al. Energy supply level correlates with ICU mortality: a multicentre study in a cohort of 1209 patients [abstract S97]. Intensive Care Med 2008. European Society for Intensive Care Medicine (ESICM), Lisbonne.
53. Woodcock NP, Zeigler D, Palmer MD, et al. Enteral versus parenteral nutrition: a pragmatic study. Nutrition 2001;17:1–12.
54. Thibault R, Heidegger CP, Methot C, et al. Supplemental Parenteral Nutrition (SPN) in ICU patients for early coverage of energy target: preliminary report. Clin Nutr 2009;4(Suppl 2):36.
55. Huang YC, Yen CE, Cheng CH, et al. Nutritional status of mechanically ventilated critically ill patients: comparison of different types of nutritional support. Clin Nutr 2000;19:101–7.
56. Bauer P, Charpentier C, Bouchet C, et al. Parenteral with enteral nutrition in the critically ill. Intensive Care Med 2000;26:893–900.

Gastric Residual Volumes in Critical Illness: What Do They Really Mean?

Ryan T. Hurt, MD[a,b,c], Stephen A. McClave, MD[d],*

KEYWORDS

• Gastric residual volumes • Enteral nutrition
• Intensive care unit • Patient outcome

The use of gastric residual volumes (GRVs) for monitoring enteral nutrition (EN) in the intensive care unit (ICU) setting is highly controversial. Despite the fact that use of GRVs is one of the most common practices in nutrition therapy, few data in the literature supports its efficacy. Although the origins of GRVs are difficult to determine, references to the practice began to appear in the nursing literature in the 1980s.[1] At the time, no data substantiated its use. No subsequent prospective randomized controlled trials suggest that their use improves patient outcomes in the ICU.[1-4] The practice of GRV monitoring was originally designed to help prevent aspiration pneumonia, yet their use serves as a major barrier to the delivery of EN in the ICU.[5] As a consequence, ironically, the use of GRVs may actually increase risk for pneumonia because of reduced delivery of EN.[6,7] Thus, although GRVs were designed to be a safeguard when delivering EN, their use may inadvertently increase risk for the patient.

Obtaining and interpreting GRVs are predicated on several assumptions. Performing GRVs assumes that the practice is well standardized, that GRVs reliably and accurately measure gastric contents, and that the practice distinguishes between normal and abnormal gastric emptying. By performing GRVs, clinicians have assumed that they are easy to interpret, that a tight correlation exists between GRVs and aspiration, and that continuing to provide EN once a high GRV above some designated level has

---

[a] Division of General Internal Medicine, Mayo Clinic, 200 1st Street SW, Rochester, MN 55905, USA
[b] Department of Medicine, University of Louisville School of Medicine, Louisville, KY, USA
[c] Department of Physiology and Biophysics, University of Louisville School of Medicine, Louisville, KY, USA
[d] Division of Gastroenterology, Hepatology, and Nutrition, University of Louisville School of Medicine, 550 South Jackson Street, Louisville, KY 40202, USA
* Corresponding author. Division of Gastroenterology, Hepatology, and Nutrition, University of Louisville School of Medicine, 550 South Jackson Street, Louisville, KY 40202.
E-mail address: samcclave@louisville.edu

Crit Care Clin 26 (2010) 481–490
doi:10.1016/j.ccc.2010.04.010   criticalcare.theclinics.com
0749-0704/10/$ – see front matter © 2010 Elsevier Inc. All rights reserved.

been reached will inadvertently lead to pneumonia and adverse outcome. And the test is assumed to be inexpensive with little or no impact on allocation of health care resources. Surprisingly, very little evidence supports any one of these assumptions. Through examining what few data support or refute each of these assumptions, clinicians should hope to reduce reliance on the practice of GRVs and alter interpretation of elevated values. This article not only reviews these assumptions but also makes recommendations for the use and interpretation of GRVs to better promote delivery of EN in patients in the ICU.

ASSUMPTION #1: THE PRACTICE OF GASTRIC RESIDUAL VOLUMES IS WELL STANDARDIZED

The practice of GRVs has numerous technical aspects, and virtually none has been well standardized in the literature. Institutions vary regarding the way in which GRVs are used clinically. Some centers use GRVs as a designated cutoff value above which cessation of tube feeds is mandated, whereas other centers use them as an initiation value below which it is appropriate to advance the rate of feeds. The absolute value for the designated cutoff value varies widely in the literature, from as little as little as 50 mL to as high as 500 mL.[7,8] Often the designated GRV may vary from one unit to the next within the same institution.[7] Still other institutions may prohibit the use of GRVs altogether. No clear consensus exists on what the appropriate GRV cutoff level should be nor how they should be used as a monitor for patients in the ICU.[5,8]

Despite whether the GRV should be discarded or reinfused back into the patient is controversial.[9,10] Simply discarding the GRV contributes to a reduced delivery of EN. In a small study from the nursing literature in which patients were randomized to have the GRV returned (n = 8) or discarded (n = 10),[10] no significant differences were seen in the rate of aspiration pneumonia, electrolyte abnormalities, need for tube replacement, or delays in feeding between the groups. In a subsequent larger single-center study of 125 patients, again randomized to have the GRV returned (n = 63) or discarded (n = 62), the severity and incidence of delayed gastric emptying was significantly lower in the group for which the GRV was returned and reinfused.[9] Intolerance measures, including diarrhea, nausea, vomiting, and abdominal distention, were no different between the groups. These two trials provide evidence supporting that GRVs below 500 mL should be routinely reinfused into the patient.[9,10]

Specific aspects of technique may alter the GRV obtained from an individual patient.[11] The size of the syringe and the material of the tubing affects the ability to obtain GRVs and the accuracy with which it measures gastric contents.[11–14] Silicone has less tensile strength than polyurethane, and therefore tubes made of silicone are more likely to collapse on aspiration. Manual aspiration with a syringe is more likely to collapse a tube than hooking the feeding tube to wall suction over several minutes. Larger-bore tubes have been shown to generate higher GRVs than smaller-bore tubes. In a study of three different sizes of tubes, Metheny and colleagues[12] showed that the mean GRV from 10-French tubes was significantly lower that the mean GRV obtained from either 14- or 18-French tubes (20.1 vs 45.8 mL, respectively; $P<.05$).

The location of the tip of the feeding tube within the gastrointestinal tract affects the GRV obtained.[15,16] Percutaneous endoscopic gastrostomy (PEG) tubes are situated on the anterior wall of the stomach. Gastric contents tend to pool in the posterior fundus when patients lies on their back, and in the antrum when they are positioned in the right lateral decubitus position. Only if the patient were in the prone position would a PEG tube be in a dependent position with regard to the gastric pool. Not surprisingly, a study comparing GRVs between PEG tubes and nasogastric tubes showed significantly lower GRVs with PEG tubes.[15] In this study, 27.4% of GRVs with a nasogastric tube were greater than 100 mL, and 15.1% were greater than 150 mL. In contrast, only 2.5% of GRVs were greater than 100 mL in patients with PEG tubes, and no GRVs were greater than 150 mL.[15] Furthermore, displacing the tip of a nasoenteric tube from the stomach to the small bowel has been shown to decrease the GRV obtained by 50%.[16]

These findings indicate that the practice of GRVs is highly variable and not standardized in any fashion. The problem for clinicians, however, is that standardizing the practice might inadvertently encourage reliance on an already inaccurate and unreliable monitor.[1,17]

ASSUMPTION #2: GASTRIC RESIDUAL VOLUMES RELIABLY AND ACCURATELY MEASURE GASTRIC CONTENTS

Based on the large volume of endogenous gastric and salivary secretions of greater than 5000 mL/d and a routine volume of EN infused between 25 and 125 mL/h, mathematical models have estimated that the GRV for gastric contents should range between 232 and 464 mL/h in patients with normal gastric emptying.[18] A critically ill patient with abnormal gastric emptying would be expected to have higher GRVs. However, two large studies evaluating GRVs in critically ill patients showed that most GRVs measured (among 90%–97% of specimens obtained) were less than 150 mL.[4,15] This disparity between the actual GRVs obtained and the volume of gastric contents that should be present suggests that the routine practice of GRVs does not accurately predict the volume of gastric contents. This disparity is further supported by the fact that 80% of the time an elevated GRV is an isolated event.[15] If GRVs accurately measured the volume of gastric contents, one would expect a more sequential pattern of elevated GRVs in response to retention and abnormalities in gastric emptying.

Knowing the location of the tip of the tube within the stomach might allow clinicians to position patients in a way that the tip would fall in a dependent position within the pool of gastric contents, yielding a more reliable GRV.[1] If the tip of the tube was known to be in the fundus, then placing the patient in the supine position would put the tip in a dependent position. If the tip were known to be in the antrum, placing the patient in the right lateral decubitus position would place the tube tip in a dependent position.[1]

Obtaining an abdominal radiograph after tube placement theoretically should then guide clinicians to the optimal patient positioning to increase reliability of GRVs. Unfortunately, at least two factors jeopardize this consideration. Even if the tube were placed in an appropriate position and the patient repositioned to accommodate this, tubes have been shown to migrate frequently back and forth within the stomach over an 8-hour period.[15] Also, when patients are placed in the supine position, the stomach drapes over the spine, causing the gastric volume to cascade into two separate pools. These two factors alone indicate that standardizing patient position for the practice of GRVs would be irrelevant.[1]

ASSUMPTION #3: GASTRIC RESIDUAL VOLUMES DISTINGUISH BETWEEN NORMAL AND ABNORMAL GASTRIC EMPTYING

Numerous factors in the ICU setting cause delayed gastric emptying (**Box 1**). Factors ranging from the clinical insult itself (eg, burns, trauma, surgery, sepsis) to those related to the nutrition therapy (eg, hypoglycemia, electrolyte abnormalities, selection of hyperosmolar formulas) may contribute to delayed gastric emptying in critically ill patients.[1] Using paracetamol absorption as a marker of gastric emptying, one study

---

Box 1
Factors in the intensive care unit that may cause decreased gastric emptying and thus affect gastric residual volumes

- Hyperglycemia
- Opiates
- Dopamine
- Increased intracranial pressure
- Electrolyte abnormalities
- Ischemia
- Hypoxia
- Sepsis
- Burns, trauma, surgery
- Hyperosmolar formulas

---

showed that patients in the ICU had a greater than threefold delay in gastric emptying compared with normal volunteers.[19] Manometric studies in critically ill patients show a virtual absence of gastric migrating motor complexes within the stomach.[20] Surprisingly though, duodenal contractions are maintained in critically ill patients. One of the benefits of early EN delivery is restoration of normal gastrointestinal physiology and the stimulation of contractility.[21,22]

An early study evaluated the accuracy with which GRVs differentiated normal from abnormal gastric emptying through comparing the practice with physical examination and abdominal radiographs.[15] A total of 26 subjects were studied over an 8-hour period, with GRVs checked every 2 hours, and a physical examination with abdominal radiograph performed at the beginning and end of the testing. Physical examination was scored for evidence of hypertimpany, abdominal distention, and hypoactive bowel sounds. The abdominal radiographs were scored for presence of air and fluid levels, dilated air-filled loops of small bowel, and gaseous distention of the stomach. Results showed that physical examination findings correlated significantly with radiographic findings ($P = .016$). However GRVs failed to correlate with either physical examination or radiographic findings.[15]

Studies directly comparing gastric emptying with GRVs have shown poor correlation. In a study again using the paracetamol absorption test as a measure of gastric emptying, Landzinski and colleagues[21] showed that in patients determined to be intolerant with high GRVs (defined by a single GRV >150 mL), 100% had abnormal gastric emptying. In contrast, of the patients determined to be tolerant with low GRVs (defined by all GRVs <150 mL), still 70% had abnormal gastric emptying.[21] In a similar fashion, Cohen and colleagues[23] showed that 25% of intolerant patients with high GRVs had normal gastric emptying, whereas Tarling and colleagues[24] showed that 57% of tolerant patients with normal GRVs had abnormal gastric emptying. These studies confirm that GRVs are inaccurate and unreliable in distinguishing normal from abnormal gastric emptying.

ASSUMPTION #4: GASTRIC RESIDUAL VOLUMES ARE EASY TO INTERPRET

The routine practice of GRVs fails to distinguish the factors that contribute to the volume of gastric contents: endogenous secretion, water flushes, and infusion of enteral formula. Although the average daily production of salivary and gastric secretions has been estimated to be as high as 3 to 5 L/d, several clinical factors exist in the ICU setting that may alter this volume.[1] Salivary output may be reduced in the absence of chewing and may be totally variable among oral, gastric, or small bowel feeding. Gastric secretion may be increased in the presence of head injury or burns, or reduced in the presence of atrophic gastritis or therapy with proton pump inhibitors. Water flushes after medication infusion, and on a regular basis to prevent clogging of the tubes, are usually poorly documented in the nursing notes. The variability in these factors alone renders the interpretation of GRVs incredibly difficult.[1]

A simple modification in the practice of GRVs, using refractometry, may improve the ease of interpretation considerably.[25] Refractometry is a standard tool to measure solute in a solution. The Brix value of a particular formula (as measured by refractometry) essentially determines the concentration of the formula, because serial dilution reduces the measurement in a linear mathematical relationship. In this manner, refractometry can be used to determine what portion of the total GRV comprises the volume of formula. The volume of formula in the stomach derived from the GRV through refractometry can then be compared with the volume of formula infused initially with the EN therapy. This alteration in the interpretation of GRVs dramatically improves interpretation of gastric emptying. A recent survey of clinicians compared data from traditional GRV with those on aspirated volume of formula determined with refractometry, obtained simultaneously in the same patients.[26] When clinicians used data from volume of formula instead of those from traditional GRVs, they were significantly more likely to interpret that the patient was having normal or even rapid gastric emptying (84% vs 33%, respectively; $P<.05$),[26] to conclude that the patient was tolerating infusion of the EN (85% vs 36%; respectively, $P<.05$), and to decide to continue the EN based on this interpretation (80% vs 34%, respectively; $P<.05$). These data suggest that traditional use of GRVs is difficult to interpret, generates false signals to suggest delayed gastric emptying, and may inadvertently lead to cessation of delivery of EN.

ASSUMPTION #5: A TIGHT CORRELATION EXISTS BETWEEN GASTRIC RESIDUAL VOLUME AND ASPIRATION

Aspiration is probably the most feared complication of EN in the ICU setting and one of the main arguments for continued use of GRV. The practice of GRVs is predicated on the assumption that a tight correlation exists between GRVs and aspiration. Although data from the literature suggest a thread of correlation between GRVs and aspiration, the relationship is tenuous at best. Therefore, for clinicians, GRVs are an inaccurate measure of risk for aspiration.

In a study using a very sensitive and specific marker for aspiration (yellow colorimetric microspheres in tracheal secretions), cutoff values for GRV ranging from 150 to 400 mL were shown to have an unacceptably low sensitivity for aspiration events of only 1.9% to 8.1%.[4] The positive predictive value of this monitor over the same range of cutoff values (the GRV above which aspiration would be expected to have occurred) was only 36.1% to 37.5%. The negative predictive value (the GRV below which no aspiration would occur) was only 70.0% to 70.3%.[4] In fact, the incidence of aspiration documented by this very sensitive and specific marker did not change over a wide range of cutoff values for GRV (from 0–50 mL to 400–500 mL).[4] Taken together, these data indicate that GRVs are a poor monitor with a very low sensitivity and specificity for detecting aspiration events in the ICU. The quality of this marker did not change by varying the cutoff value for GRV from 150 to 400 mL.[4]

Nonetheless, two other studies using a different marker for aspiration showed a thread of correlation between GRVs and aspiration.[14,27] Using the presence of pepsin in tracheal secretions as a surrogate marker of aspiration, patients with a high frequency of aspiration were shown to be more likely to have GRVs greater than 200 mL than those with a low frequency of aspiration (75% incidence of GRVs >200 mL vs 25%, respectively; $P = .08$).[27] In a second study using the same marker, Metheny and colleagues[14] showed that when high GRVs were present, the risk of aspiration increased significantly. However, in both studies, results showed no significant correlation between GRVs and aspiration when specifically evaluated.[14,27]

ASSUMPTION #6: CONTINUING ENTERAL NUTRITION AFTER OBTAINING A HIGH GASTRIC RESIDUAL VOLUME LEADS TO PNEUMONIA AND ADVERSE OUTCOME

Despite whether aspiration is involved as the mediating event, another key assumption made when practicing GRVs is that continuing to provide EN after a high GRV has been obtained will lead to pneumonia and other adverse patient outcomes. Again, scant evidence from the literature suggests a thread of correlation between high GRVs and pneumonia. In a study by Mentec and colleagues,[13] GRVs alone correlated with increased sedation, use of catecholamines (as pressor agents), and reduced caloric intake. When GRVs were combined with vomiting to define "upper digestive intolerance," that combination of events correlated significantly to pneumonia, ICU length of stay, and ICU mortality.[13] Closer evaluation of the data, however, showed that GRVs alone did not correlate with ICU mortality, hospital mortality, or incidence of pneumonia.[13]

This particular assumption, however, has led clinicians to fear that increasing the cutoff value for GRV will lead to increased aspiration and pneumonia. Conversely, through self-assurance, clinicians believe that decreasing the value will actually protect patients against aspiration and pneumonia. Data from four prospective controlled trials randomizing patients to two different cutoff levels for GRV show that these beliefs are baseless.[4,6,28,29]

In a study by Taylor and colleagues,[6] patients randomized to a 200-mL cutoff value for GRV received a significantly greater percentage of goal calories than those randomized to a 150-mL cutoff value (59% of goal calories vs 36%, respectively; $P<.05$). Similarly, in a study by Montejo and colleagues,[29] patients randomized to a 500-mL cutoff value for GRV received a significantly greater percentage of goal calories than those randomized to a 200-mL cutoff value (89% vs 83%, respectively; $P<.05$).

In a study randomizing patients to 150 versus 250 mL for the cutoff value for GRVs, Pinilla and colleagues[28] found that the incidence of vomiting and gastrointestinal intolerance was no different between groups. In a study from Louisville, randomizing patients to 200 versus 400 mL as the cutoff value for GRVs, the incidence of regurgitation and aspiration were the same between the groups.[4]

Remarkably, in the study by Taylor and colleagues,[6] patients randomized to 150 mL GRV had significantly higher overall complications than the group randomized to 200 mL (61% vs 37%, respectively; $P<.05$). In the Montejo and colleagues[29] study, gastrointestinal complications were higher in the patients randomized to 200 mL GRV than in those randomized to 500 mL (63.6% vs 47.8%, respectively; $P<.05$).

In fact, two additional studies have evaluated the impact on patient outcome of eliminating the practice of GRVs altogether.[30,31] In a small nursing study by Powell and colleagues,[30] the incidence of aspiration pneumonia was no different between study patients in whom no residual volumes were used and controls in whom routine use of GRVs was performed. The incidence of tube clogging, however, was reduced 10-fold in the study patients in whom GRVs were not used (7.7% incidence vs 66.7% in controls; $P<.05$).[30] In a second prospective before-and-after study, patients for whom no GRVs were used had a lower incidence of intolerance, a higher volume of EN infused, and no difference in vomiting or ventilator-associated pneumonia compared with controls in whom routine GRVs were performed.[31]

Further irony regarding this assumption that continuing EN after a high GRV or raising the cutoff value for GRV will lead to pneumonia and adverse outcome is the fact that the use of GRVs often leads to inappropriate cessation of EN, and the risk for subsequent pneumonia may actually increase. In a study by Meissner and colleagues,[32] a narcotic antagonist was infused through the feeding tube to patients on mechanical ventilation receiving fentanyl to promote gastrointestinal motility. Greater contractility in study patients led to a greater volume of EN infused (1200 vs 1000 mL, respectively; $P<.05$) and a significant reduction in the incidence of pneumonia (36% vs 55%, respectively; $P<.05$) compared with controls who received placebo.[32] In the study by Taylor and colleagues,[6] patients randomized to the protocol with a higher cutoff value for GRV and who received nearly twice the volume of EN had a significant reduction in the incidence of infection (85% vs 61%, respectively; $P<.05$) and a nonsignificant reduction in the incidence of pneumonia (63% vs 44%, respectively) compared with controls.

These data suggest that a tenuous yet unreliable relationship exists among GRVs, aspiration, and pneumonia. In an effort to protect patients through use of GRVs, clinicians may inadvertently cause more frequent cessation of EN and the risk of pneumonia may actually increase. Changing the cutoff level for GRVs does nothing to improve the accuracy or predictability of GRVs as a marker for aspiration or pneumonia. The failure of GRVs to accurately predict aspiration or pneumonia precludes reliance on this monitor in the critical care setting.

ASSUMPTION #7: GASTRIC RESIDUAL VOLUMES ARE AN INEXPENSIVE "POOR MAN'S TEST" FOR GASTRIC EMPTYING AND TOLERANCE OF ENTERAL NUTRITION

When performing GRVs, most clinicians assume the practice is an inexpensive, simplistic method for gauging tolerance for EN and gastric emptying. However, every nursing duty in the ICU represents an allocation of health care resources. Parrish and McClave[1] showed that a nurse spends an average of 5.25 minutes performing GRV tests. Thus, the allocation of health care resources (in 2006 U.S. dollars) for a nurse on a median salary to perform GRVs on 100 patients (every 4 hours for a 3-day average ICU length of stay) would be $453,600.[1] This cost represents a significant allocation of resources for a monitor that is inaccurate and unreliable. This time might be better spent elevating the head of the bed, providing good oral hygiene, developing and enforcing an EN protocol, or calculating and readjusting volume-based feeds to make up for lost time required for diagnostic tests.

SUMMARY

Despite the fallacies of every one of the assumptions made when performing GRVs, clinicians are unlikely to stop performing this routine test in the ICU. Therefore, efficacy of EN therapy can only improve if clinicians are able to modify their response to and interpretation of GRVs (**Box 2**).[1]

Clinicians may continue to check GRVs every 4 hours after initiation of EN, being careful to return aspirated contents less than 500 mL to the patient. In the absence of other signs of intolerance, stopping the delivery of EN for any GRV less than 400

> **Box 2**
> **Summary of recommendations for using gastric residual volumes in an enteral nutrition protocol**
>
> - Check GRV every 4 hours
> - Return contents to patient if less than 500 mL
> - If first GRV greater than 400 mL, initiate the following:
>   1. Continue EN at the current rate
>   2. Turn patient to the right lateral decubitus position if possible for 30 minutes
>   3. Begin reglan, 10 mg, intravenously, every 6 hours
>   4. Begin narcan, 8 mg, in 10 mL of saline through feeding tube every 6 hours
>   5. Recheck GRV in 4 hours
> - Only if second consecutive GRV 4 hours later is greater than 400 mL, hold EN and:
>   1. Recheck GRV every 2 hours, restart EN when GRV is less than 400 mL
>   2. If no signs of intolerance, restart at same rate
>   3. If evidence of intolerance present, consider reducing rate by 25 mL/h or to baseline of 25 mL/h

to 500 mL is inappropriate. For the first GRV greater than 400 mL, EN should be continued at its current rate, the patient should be turned over to the right lateral decubitus position (to put the antrum in the dependent position and promote gastric emptying), and prokinetic therapy with metoclopramide, 10 mg, should be initiated intravenously every 6 hours. If the patient is on opioid narcotics, clinicians could consider an infusion of naloxone, 8 mg, in 10 mL of saline through the feeding tube every 6 hours. If a second GRV 4 hours later is greater than 400 mL, then holding EN while the patient is being reassessed may be appropriate. GRVs should be rechecked every 2 hours at that point, with EN restarted once the GRV drops to less than 400 mL. If no other signs of tolerance are present, the EN may be started at the same rate. If other signs of intolerance are present (eg, abdominal distention, hypoactive bowel sounds, failure to pass stool or gas), then reducing the rate by 25 mL/h or to a baseline of 25 mL/h may be wise. Checking GRVs is more important on initiation of EN. Once EN has been infused successfully for 48 to 72 hours, clinicians should be encouraged to stop checking GRVs and simply follow physical findings for any clinical signs of intolerance.[1]

Early and adequate delivery of EN has been linked to improved patient outcomes. EN therapy in critically ill patients in the ICU is difficult, and excessive emphasis on GRVs tends to impede its delivery. The current use of GRVs is based on several flawed assumptions with little scientific basis. GRVs should never be interpreted in a vacuum, without paying attention to signs on physical examination of intolerance and intestinal ileus. Having protocols in place improves the interpretation and response to elevated GRVs, reduces inappropriate cessation, and promotes a greater percentage of goal calories of EN delivered. Once tolerance of EN is established, ceasing the performance of GRVs may be appropriate to better allocate nursing time and health care resources.

REFERENCES

1. Parrish RP, McClave SA. Checking gastric residual volumes: a practice in search of science? Pract Gastroenterol 2008;32(10):33–47.

2. McClave SA, Dryden GW. Critical care nutrition: reducing the risk of aspiration. Semin Gastrointest Dis 2003;14(1):2–10.
3. Elpern EH, Stutz L, Peterson S, et al. Outcomes associated with enteral tube feedings in a medical intensive care unit. Am J Crit Care 2004;13(3):221–7.
4. McClave SA, Lukan JK, Stefater JA, et al. Poor validity of residual volumes as a marker for risk of aspiration in critically ill patients. Crit Care Med 2005;33(2): 324–30.
5. Poulard F, Dimet J, Martin-Lefevre L, et al. Impact of not measuring residual gastric volume in mechanically ventilated patients receiving early enteral feeding: a prospective before-after study. JPEN J Parenter Enteral Nutr 2010;34(2): 125–30.
6. Taylor SJ, Fettes SB, Jewkes C, et al. Prospective, randomized, controlled trial to determine the effect of early enhanced enteral nutrition on clinical outcome in mechanically ventilated patients suffering head injury. Crit Care Med 1999;27(11): 2525–31.
7. Adam S, Batson S. A study of problems associated with the delivery of enteral feed in critically ill patients in five ICUs in the UK. Intensive Care Med 1997; 23(3):261–6.
8. Edwards SJ, Metheny NA. Measurement of gastric residual volume: state of the science. Medsurg Nurs 2000;9(3):125–8.
9. Juve-Udina ME, Valls-Miró C, Carreño-Granero A, et al. To return or to discard? Randomised trial on gastric residual volume management. Intensive Crit Care Nurs 2009;25(5):258–67.
10. Booker KJ, Niedringhaus L, Eden B, et al. Comparison of 2 methods of managing gastric residual volumes from feeding tubes. Am J Crit Care 2000;9(5):318–24.
11. Metheny N, Reed L, Worseck M, et al. How to aspirate fluid from small-bore feeding tubes. Am J Nurs 1993;93(5):86–8.
12. Metheny NA, Stewart J, Nuetzel G, et al. Effect of feeding-tube properties on residual volume measurements in tube-fed patients. JPEN J Parenter Enteral Nutr 2005;29(3):192–7.
13. Mentec H, Dupont H, Bocchetti M, et al. Upper digestive intolerance during enteral nutrition in critically ill patients: frequency, risk factors, and complications. Crit Care Med 2001;29(10):1955–61.
14. Metheny NA, Schallom L, Oliver DA, et al. Gastric residual volume and aspiration in critically ill patients receiving gastric feedings. Am J Crit Care 2008;17(6): 512–9 [quiz: 520].
15. McClave SA, Snider HL, Lowen CC, et al. Use of residual volume as a marker for enteral feeding intolerance: prospective blinded comparison with physical examination and radiographic findings. JPEN J Parenter Enteral Nutr 1992;16(2):99–105.
16. Esparza J, Boivin MA, Hartshorne MF, et al. Equal aspiration rates in gastrically and transpylorically fed critically ill patients. Intensive Care Med 2001;27(4): 660–4.
17. Metheny NA. Residual volume measurement should be retained in enteral feeding protocols. Am J Crit Care 2008;17(1):62–4.
18. Lin HC, Van Citters GW. Stopping enteral feeding for arbitrary gastric residual volume may not be physiologically sound: results of a computer simulation model. JPEN J Parenter Enteral Nutr 1997;21(5):286–9.
19. Heyland DK, Tougas G, King D, et al. Impaired gastric emptying in mechanically ventilated, critically ill patients. Intensive Care Med 1996;22(12):1339–44.
20. Dive A, Moulart M, Jonard P, et al. Gastroduodenal motility in mechanically ventilated critically ill patients: a manometric study. Crit Care Med 1994;22(3):441–7.

21. Landzinski J, Kiser TH, Fish DN, et al. Gastric motility function in critically ill patients tolerant vs intolerant to gastric nutrition. JPEN J Parenter Enteral Nutr 2008;32(1):45–50.

22. Kompan L, Kremzar B, Gadzijev E, et al. Effects of early enteral nutrition on intestinal permeability and the development of multiple organ failure after multiple injury. Intensive Care Med 1999;25(2):157–61.

23. Cohen J, Aharon A, Singer P. The paracetamol absorption test: a useful addition to the enteral nutrition algorithm. Clin Nutr 2000;19:233–6.

24. Tarling MM, Toner CC, Withington PS, et al. A model of gastric emptying using paracetamol absorbtion in intensive care patients. Intensive Care Med 1997;23: 256–9.

25. Chang WK, McClave SA, Chao YC. Enhancing interpretation of gastric residual volume by refractometry. Nutr Clin Pract 2004;19:455–62.

26. McClave SA, Chang WK, Mikola D, et al. Use of refractometry to determine volume of formula remaining in the stomach improves interpretation of gastric residual volume and facilitates delivery of enteral nutrition. JPEN 2009;33(2):223.

27. Metheny NA, Clouse RE, Chang YH, et al. Tracheobronchial aspiration of gastric contents in critically ill tube-fed patients: frequency, outcomes, and risk factors. Crit Care Med 2006;34(4):1007–15.

28. Pinilla JC, Samphire J, Arnold C, et al. Comparison of gastrointestinal tolerance to two enteral feeding protocols in critically ill patients: a prospective, randomized controlled trial. JPEN J Parenter Enteral Nutr 2001;25(2):81–6.

29. Montejo-Gonzales JC, Minambres E, Bordeje L, et al. Gastric residual volume during enteral nutrition in ICU patients. The REGANE study. Preliminary results [abstract]. Intensive Care Med 2007;33(Suppl 2):S108.

30. Powell KS, Marcuard SP, Farrior ES, et al. Aspirating gastric residuals causes occlusion of small-bore feeding tubes. J Parenter Enteral Nutr 1993;17:243–6.

31. Poulard F, Dimet J, Martin-Lefevre L, et al. Impact of not measuring gastric residual volume in mechanically ventilated patients receiving early enteral feeding: a prospective before-after study. JPEN 2010;34(2):125–30.

32. Meissner W, Dohrn B, Reinhart K. Enteral naloxone reduces gastric tube reflux and frequency of pneumonia in critical care patients during opioid analgesia. Crit Care Med 2003;31(3):776–80.

Immunosupression and Infection After Major Surgery: A Nutritional Deficiency

Xinmei Zhu, MD, PhD, Gabriel Herrera, MD, Juan B. Ochoa, MD*

KEYWORDS

- T cell dysfunction • Immunosuppression • Nutrition deficiency
- Arginine • Arginine deficiency syndrome

Infection after surgery and trauma (or major physical injury [PI]) is a central cause for increased morbidity, mortality, and cost. Alterations in both innate and adaptive immune function contribute significantly to increased susceptibility to infections. This in turn leads to the development of organ failure and death. Of the many alterations reported, adaptive T cell dysfunction is consistently observed at the bedside and in animal models of PI, and it is thought to increase the risk of infection.[1] It follows that understanding why trauma and surgical patients are susceptible to infections should lead to the development of successful treatment.

Diets containing supraphysiologic quantities or arginine, omega 3 fatty acids, nucleotides, and antioxidants were developed over 25 years ago.[2] These diets were called immune-enhancing diets (IEDs), a name that remains in the literature up until today. These diets have been tested in multiple studies, mostly in critically ill and surgical patients. IEDs improve T helper cell (CD4+) counts and may increase NO production, and they are associated with a significant and consistent decrease the risk of infection in patients undergoing major elective surgery.[3,4] The use of IEDs in medical critically ill patients and in patients with sepsis is far more controversial. In these populations, no clear benefit has been observed.[5] To date, IEDs remain the only effective therapy that restores immune function and decreases infection rates after PI.

The mechanisms of how these diets exert their effect have been unknown until recently. New advances, however, have led to a series of fascinating discoveries as to how the control of arginine availability by the immune system has evolved as a major

Funding: Grant # NIH- MIGMS–065914
F1264 PUH-UPMC, 200 Lothrop Street, Pittsburgh, PA 15213, USA
* Corresponding author.
E-mail address: ochoajb@upmc.edu

Crit Care Clin 26 (2010) 491–500
doi:10.1016/j.ccc.2010.04.004   criticalcare.theclinics.com

regulatory mechanism with important biologic roles.[6] This article describes arginine starvation as a mechanism of immune control.[7]

ARGININE DEFICIENCY IS OBSERVED AFTER PI

That arginine becomes deficient after PI is a well-described fact. Arginine was discovered over 100 years ago, and is a basic, nonessential amino acid, naturally ingested at a rate of approximately 3 to 5 g/d. Studies in the first part of the 20th century demonstrated that arginine was necessary for growth.[8,9] This also was reported in 1978 by Seifter and colleagues[10] and confirmed by Wakabayashi and colleagues[11] in 1994. Serendipitous observations led to the discovery that arginine prevented thymic involution after injury and appeared to play a critical role in maintaining T lymphocyte function.[12] Moreover, arginine was found to be necessary for adequate wound healing. Thus, an initial classification of arginine as a semiessential amino acid was given. Some investigators even summarized these observations in the statement that arginine was a "conditionally essential amino acid," which should be supplemented at times of physical stress such as after surgery, trauma, or growth.

Within hours after PI, arginine plasma levels drop by 50% or more and remain depressed for days or weeks (**Fig. 1**).[13] The drop in plasma arginine appears to be resistant to dietary supplementation even when given at supraphysiologic concentrations. For example, Tsuei and colleagues[14] provided 30 g of daily enteral arginine intake to trauma patients starting within 24 hours after injury. Despite successfully delivering this amount, arginine plasma levels failed to improve for the first 5 days, reaching only a statistically significant increase in plasma arginine by day 7. In contrast, ornithine plasma levels increase significantly after the first arginine dose, suggesting that PI induces alternative arginine-metabolizing enzymes.

ARGININE DEFICIENCY AFFECTS BIOLOGIC FUNCTIONS

A decrease in arginine plasma levels does not guarantee that a state of arginine deficiency exists. In fact, if arginine-dependant processes were not affected, arginine plasma levels would be of no significance. The authors have evaluated two arginine-dependent processes: nitric oxide production and T lymphocyte function. Significant data have accumulated to demonstrate that both biologic functions are

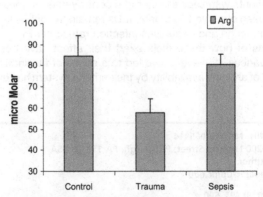

Fig. 1. Arginine plasma levels drop significantly after physical injury (major trauma). In contrast, arginine plasma levels were similar in the control group and in septic patients.

profoundly affected after PI. The mechanisms that explain these phenomena are discussed.

NO Production

Arginine is the sole amino acid substrate for the production of NO. NO is produced by multiple cell types and by three different isoenzymes. Endothelial NO synthase (eNOS) plays an important role in vasodilation and microcirculation. NO synthase can be induced (iNOS) in myeloid cells, hepatocytes, and other cell types and plays an important role in immune responses. Finally, neuronal NO synthase (nNOS) may play important roles in complex central nervous system functions.[8]

In 1991, the authors first reported the accumulation of NO metabolites (mainly nitrates, NO_3^-) in septic and trauma patients. Nitrates accumulated in septic patients but did not accumulate after trauma even when they became septic. Further evaluation of this phenomenon demonstrated that the urinary excretion of NO_3^- also was decreased significantly.[15] To further study this, the authors developed a rodent model of moderate trauma by performing a laparotomy under anesthesia (**Fig. 2**). Similar to people, rodents after injury failed to accumulate NO_3^- in plasma even after receiving endotoxin (**Fig. 3**). In a similar way, mice subjected to surgical injury also exhibit a decrease in circulating arginine. The authors have exploited this model to further study of arginine metabolism after PI.

Work performed by several investigators has demonstrated that arginine supplementation after injury leads to an increase in circulating NO metabolites and evidence of improved microcirculation. For example, the use of arginine supplementation led to the accumulation of NO metabolites in local wound flaps created in pigs and significantly increased flap viability.[16] Independent research performed by Tepaske and colleagues[4] in patients undergoing open heart surgery and receiving an oral dietary supplement containing supraphysiologic arginine concentrations led to decreased accumulation of base deficit in lactate (evidence of improved microcirculation) within the first 24 hours after the surgical procedure. Evidence therefore points to the fact that a decrease in circulating arginine in plasma after injury also leads to decreased production of NO.

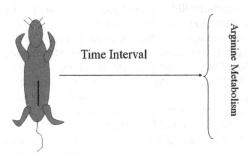

Exploratory Laparotomy

Fig. 2. A rodent model of moderate physical injury (PI) has served as an important tool with which to study arginine metabolism. In this model, PI is induced by performing an exploratory laparotomy under anesthesia. After opening the abdomen, the bowel is manipulated gently. The severity of PI can be altered by either leaving the abdomen open or by the length of bowel manipulated. The abdomen then is closed in two layers. Most animals survive this insult but may require some crystalloid resuscitation. Arginine metabolism using this model can be studied in any tissue and has been studied extensively in plasma and the spleen.

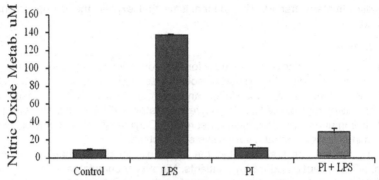

Fig. 3. Accumulation of nitric oxide metabolites in plasma after PI in rodents. Mice were subjected to PI (see **Fig. 2**). 24 hours later, some of the mice received endotoxin (LPS) (5 mg/kg) IP. Control mice were not subjected to PI and did not receive endotoxin. Yet another group received endotoxin but were not subjected to PI. Accumulation of NO metabolites was observed in plasma after endotoxin in the absence of PI but was not observed in mice subjected to PI even when endotoxin was given (PI + LPS). (*From* Munera V, Popovic PJ, Bryk J, et al. Stat 6-dependent induction of myeloid derived suppressor cells after physical injury regulates nitric oxide response to endotoxin. Ann Surg 2010;251:120–6; with permission.)

T Lymphocyte Function

T lymphocytes depend on arginine for normal function and proliferation; therefore studying T lymphocytes provides an important target to test the hypothesis that arginine deficiency develops after injury. The authors created an in vitro model where mouse T lymphocytes were cultured in the presence of different concentrations of arginine ranging from supraphysiologic concentrations (1000 µM) to severely deficient arginine levels (<10 µM). Of note, normal plasma arginine levels are approximately 80 to 120 µM. T cell proliferation was proportional to the concentration of arginine but reached a plateau at 100 µM arginine levels. Both CD4+ and CD8+ were sensitive to arginine depletion (**Fig. 4**). Interleukin (IL)-2 was modestly sensitive to arginine depletion.[17,18] Other investigators, using similar models, have reported similar observations for other cytokines (interferon [IFN]- γ and IL-4).[19] In addition, cells cultured in arginine-deficient media appeared to be unable to develop into memory T lymphocytes. It also was noticed that the membrane concentration of the CD3 receptor complex was directly proportional to the concentration of arginine in the culture media. The authors therefore tested the effect of arginine concentrations on expression of the different peptides forming the T cell receptor (TCR) complex including that of the ζ chain. TCR integrity is vital for the induction of optimal and efficient immune responses, including the routine elimination of invading pathogens and the elimination of modified cells and molecules. The subunit of TCR, CD3 z-chain, is the main signal–transduction component of the TCR and is required for correct assembly of the receptor complex. Interestingly, ζ chain expression was exquisitely sensitive to arginine deprivation and presently remains a significant biomarker of arginine deficiency.[20,21]

T lymphocyte dysfunction after PI is characterized by decreased T cell proliferation, anergic responses to antigen recall, decreased IL-2 and IFN γ production, and loss of ζ chain; these findings are remarkably similar to those observed when T lymphocytes are cultured in arginine-deficient media. Several other diseases are associated with T lymphocyte dysfunction and loss of the ζ chain, including renal cell carcinoma, tuberculosis, and leprosy.[22] Similar to that observed after PI, these diseases may be associated with a decrease in plasma arginine levels.[23] Thus, accumulating evidence

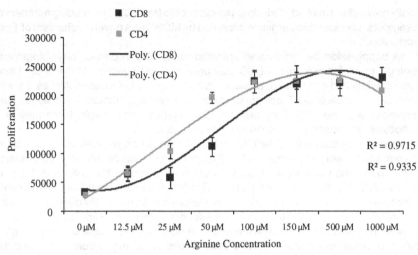

Fig. 4. Effect of arginine on T cell proliferation to antigenic stimuli (anti-CD3/anti-CD28). T cell subpopulations (CD4, CD8), were separated and placed in culture in increasing concentration of arginine (0 to 1000 μM). Cell proliferation was measured using ^{3}H-thymidine incorporation after 48 hours in culture. Proliferation of T lymphocyte subpopulations was proportional to arginine up to 100 μM. Increasing arginine above this level did not increase T cell proliferation. Regression analysis demonstrated an $R^2 > .9$ for both supopulations. (*From* Ochoa JB, Strange J, Kearney P, et al. Effects of L-arginine on the proliferation of T lymphocyte subpopulations. JPEN J Parenter Enteral Nutr 2001;25:23–9; with permission.)

demonstrates that a decrease in circulating arginine after PI is also associated with characteristic alterations in accumulation of NO metabolites and T lymphocyte function. These observations are therefore supportive of the hypothesis that PI induces a state of arginine deficiency.

MYELOID CELLS AFTER PI EXPRESS ARGINASE 1 AND DEPLETE ARGININE

A decrease in circulating arginine is evident within a few hours after injury. This observation argues that arginine deficiency does not develop from lack of intake, but rather through increased destruction. Arginase 1 (ARG1), like iNOS, is an inducible enzyme in myeloid cells. ARG1 metabolizes arginine to ornithine and urea. The hypothesis that ARG1 was induced after physical injury in myeloid cells was tested in the mouse model of surgical trauma previously described. A progressive induction of ARG1 expression along with an increase in arginase activity was detected in splenic tissues. These initial observations led to the identification that ARG1 expression was exclusively localized to myeloid cells that accumulated in large numbers within hours of injury.[24] Cultured myeloid cells expressing ARG1 demonstrate depletion of arginine and accumulation of ornithine in the culture media. PI-induced myeloid cells expressing ARG1 are therefore capable of creating a state of arginine depletion. These cells exhibit a granulocyte-like appearance, and are immature cells as evidenced by their expression of GR1; they also rapidly accumulate in the marginal zones in the spleen, virtually surrounding T lymphocytes.

When placed in culture with T lymphocytes, immature myeloid cells expressing ARG1 inhibit T lymphocyte growth and function. T cell function is restored when supraphysiologic quantities of arginine are added to the culture media or ARG1 is pharmacologically inhibited. Hence, myeloid cells induced by PI become immunosuppressor cells and are officially now called myeloid-derived suppressor cells (MDSC).[25] Increasing numbers of investigators have identified arginine depletion by MDSC as a novel mechanism of T cell suppression.

T cell suppression by amino acid starvation may play important physiologic and pathologic roles; for example, MDSC may prevent T cell rejection of the fetus during pregnancy. Myeloid-derived suppressor cells are rapidly being accepted as a major mechanism of pathologic T cell suppression in a growing number of illnesses. Not surprisingly, arginine deficiency and the characteristic phenotypical changes in T lymphocytes are observed in these disease processes.

The common features to all MDSCs are their myeloid origin, their immature state, and a remarkable ability to suppress T-cell responses.[26] Actually, MDSCs are a heterogeneous population of cells that consists of myeloid progenitor cells and IMCs. In healthy individuals, IMCs that are generated in the bone marrow quickly differentiate into mature granulocytes, macrophages, or dendritic cells (DCs). By contrast, in pathologic conditions such as cancer, various infectious diseases, sepsis, trauma, bone marrow transplantation, and some autoimmune diseases, a partial block in the differentiation of IMCs into mature myeloid cells results in the expansion of this population.[27] Thus, MDSCs are normally found in low numbers in lymphoid organs. In an inflammatory environment, however, the accumulation of regulatory MDSCs has been detected in lymphoid organs during tumor growth.

OVERCOMING ARGININE DEPLETION BY MDSC

The identification of a novel mechanism of T cell suppression and decreased NO production through arginine depletion by MDSC opens a significant opportunity for treatment not only in surgical patients but in other disease processes also. Several strategies are being proposed in the literature. The first strategy would be to block the induction of MDSC or upregulation of ARG1 expression.[20] Several investigators have delineated the messages that induced the expression of MDSC and ARG1. These include T2 helper messages such as IL-4/IL-13, catecholamines, and prostaglandins.[28–30] Particular attention has been placed to prostaglandin E2 (PGE2), as it seems to be an important messenger released by tumors to recruit MDSCs.

Our group tested the effect of different prostaglandins on the induction of ARG1 in the presence or absence of IL-13 in RAW 264.7 cells, a myeloid cell line.[31,32] This study focused on the fact that the type of fatty acid supplementation is associated with the production of different prostaglandins. Thus, for example, borage oil supplementation will preferentially lead to the formation of PGE1, while PGE2 is produced from corn oil, and PGE3 is generated from fish oil. All prostaglandins induced ARG1 and synergized with IL-13. The degree of ARG1 induction was significantly different, however, with evident blunting observed for PGE3 when compared with PGE1 or PGE2. NO production was inversely proportional to the induction of ARG1, again demonstrating that arginase could block iNOS through competition for the available arginine. Studies performed by independent investigators also demonstrate that fish oil supplementation may blunt the upregulation of CD16+ cells in people; this finding corresponds to the MDSC observed in mice.[33] Thus the summary of these studies demonstrates a proof of concept that the addition of fish oil to a diet potentially serves to prevent the upregulation of MDSC and ARG1 expression.

A second dietary strategy is to overcome arginine deficiency with the supplementation of supraphysiologic quantities of the amino acid itself. Arginine can be administered orally at increased concentrations of up to 30 g/d, although there may be significant intestinal adverse effects including nausea, bloating, and diarrhea.

Supraphysiologic dietary arginine intake significantly increases arginine plasma levels and arginine availability and thus may help in overcoming arginine deficiency caused by MDSC.

Yet another dietary strategy is that of inducing the maturation of MDSCs. Myeloid-derived suppressor cells can mature into granulocytes, dendritic cells, or macrophages.[34] Interestingly, all-trans retinoic acids (ATRA, part of the vitamin A family of compounds) promote maturation of MDSC into specific myeloid cell lineages. Of note, mature myeloid cells loose their capacity to suppress T cell function. ATRA is being tested in prospective randomized trials in patients with cancer to determine its effect on maturation of MDSC and improvement of T cell function.

It would be ideal that each individual component of a diet could and would be tested separately in the same manner that a pharmacologic agent is tested.[35,36] This may not be practical, however, or even possible. Thus, most studies test the effect of a diet containing several different nutrients at the same time.

CLINICAL STUDIES OF DIETARY ARGININE SUPPLEMENTATION

Starting from 1980s, some animal experiments suggested that arginine could have beneficial effects in restoring T lymphocyte counts under conditions of stress. Based on these observations, commercial diets were created to enhance immunity and hopefully prevent or decrease the severity of infections. The amount of arginine added was significantly higher than that of the normal dietary intake, ranging from 8 to 30 g/d. In most of the trials, arginine has been added to other nutrients with immune activity such as omega-3 fatty acids, nucleotides, and vitamin A; hence the name immune-enhancing diets (IEDs). To date more than 40 trials using IEDs have been performed in a wide variety of patient populations. These trials demonstrate a consistent benefit by reducing infections in patients undergoing high-risk surgery.[35,36] Interestingly, the benefits observed in surgical patients appear not to be present in medical critically ill patients or in patients with primary sepsis, diseases that are not necessarily associated with decreased arginine availability.

Several of these studies are worth reviewing in more detail. In 2002, Braga and Gianotti and others reported a prospective randomized trial testing a dietary supplement that contained arginine (12.5 g/L) and omega 3 fatty acids (3.3 g/L). This trial was done exclusively in patients with histologically proven colon cancer electively scheduled to undergo colon resection. Patients were randomized into four different groups as follows:

1. A preoperative group that received the experimental diet before surgery but a conventional management postoperatively
2. A perioperative group that received the experimental diet both before and after surgery
3. A control group that received an isonitrogenous oral dietary supplement
4. A conventional group that received no dietary supplements.

The investigators tested several endpoints, including immune parameters, microperfusion of the colon, and outcomes. Fifty patients were admitted to each group on an intent-to-treat basis. Patients receiving preoperative dietary supplements exhibited significant improvements in delayed-type hypersensitivity postoperatively, a decrease in IL-6 levels, improved colonic microprofusion, and a significant decrease in infection rates and antibiotic use, along with shorter length of stay.[37,38]

Tepaske reported a prospective randomized trial, that similar to Braga's work, tested the use of an experimental diet in 25 patients containing arginine and omega

3 fatty acids. Twenty-five additional patients were used as controls. All patients underwent open-heart surgery. Patients receiving the experimental diet exhibited decreased accumulation of lactate and base deficit (suggesting improved microcirculation), improvement in delayed-type hypersensitivity, and an overall significant decrease in infection rates.[4]

Trauma patients also appear to benefit from these diets, but they must be started soon (ideally within 24 hours) after injury. Kudsk and colleagues prospectively randomized patients with severe trauma to receive a diet containing arginine and omega 3 fatty acids (n = 17) or receive an isonitrogenous, isocaloric enteral diet (n = 18). Six percent of patients receiving an enteral diet developed infectious complications as opposed to 41% of those on a conventional diet who developed infectious complications (P = .002). To date, this study remains one of the best prospective randomized trials in immunonutrition.[39]

The use of IEDs in critically ill medical (nonsurgical) patients has been far more controversial. Concerning is the fact that in some of these studies, mixed results have been observed in septic critically ill patients, with some studies describing increased mortality, whereas others report the opposite result. These uncertain results make the use of IED highly controversial in sepsis.[5]

The critical components of IEDs and how they interact with each other remain unknown. In an effort to determine interactions between these nutrients, the authors' laboratory has done some preliminary studies that demonstrate that prostaglandins (derived from omega-3 fatty acids) can increase available arginine by decreasing ARG1 expression. Thus, the specific combinations of dietary fatty acids and arginine should be considered when tailoring dietary regimens.

WRAPPING IT ALL UP—ARGININE DEFICIENCY SYNDROME

The authors propose that arginine deficiency after PI is an important clinical syndrome, as there are clinically characteristic signs and symptoms that are related to the decreased arginine availability.[6] Arginine deficiency after PI produces characteristic changes in T lymphocyte function and NO production. Myeloid-derived suppressor cells are capable of metabolizing arginine into ornithine and urea and depleting arginine from the surrounding environment. In addition, the authors have identified the mechanisms that lead to the upregulation of MDSC and ARG1. Arginine deficiency caused by MDSC can be treated via dietary supplementation. Finally, multiple clinical studies demonstrate that treatment with diets containing supraphysiologic concentrations of arginine along with omega 3 fatty acids and potentially other nutrients restores immune function and prevents infections.

It should be possible to provide an early identification of arginine deficiency syndrome in a growing number of illnesses including cancer, leprosy, tuberculosis, and other diseases. Early treatment of arginine deficiency syndrome should lead to improvement in prognosis and outcomes in these illnesses. Arginine deficiency syndrome is probably already empirically being treated with the use of IEDs in surgical and trauma patients. The use of IEDs in patients undergoing major surgical should become standard of care, as its use decreases infections and cost in this patient population.

REFERENCES

1. Mannick JA, Rodrick ML, Lederer JA. The immunologic response to injury. J Am Coll Surg 2001;193:237–44.
2. Beale RJ, Bryg DJ, Bihari DJ. Immunonutrition in the critically ill: a systematic review of clinical outcome. Crit Care Med 1999;27:2799–805.

3. Daly JM, Lieberman MD, Goldfine J, et al. Enteral nutrition with supplemental arginine, RNA, and omega-3 fatty acids in patients after operation: immunologic, metabolic, and clinical outcome. Surgery 1992;112:56–67.
4. Tepaske R, Velthuis H, Oudemans-van Straaten HM, et al. Effect of preoperative oral immune-enhancing nutritional supplement on patients at high risk of infection after cardiac surgery: a randomised placebo-controlled trial. Lancet 2001;358:696–701.
5. Heyland DK, Novak F, Drover JW, et al. Should immunonutrition become routine in critically ill patients? A systematic review of the evidence. JAMA 2001;286:944–53.
6. Popovic PJ, Zeh HJ III, Ochoa JB. Arginine and immunity. J Nutr 2007;137: 1681S–6.
7. Bronte V, Serafini P, Mazzoni A, et al. L-arginine metabolism in myeloid cells controls T-lymphocyte functions. Trends Immunol 2003;24:302–6.
8. Morris SM Jr. Regulation of arginine availability and its impact on NO synthesis. In: Ignarro LJ, editor. Nitric oxide: biology and pathobiology. San Diego (CA): Academic Press; 2000. p. 187–97.
9. Morris SM Jr. Arginine: beyond protein. Am J Clin Nutr 2006;83:508S–12.
10. Seifter E, Rettura G, Barbul A, et al. Arginine: an essential amino acid for injured rats. Surgery 1978;84:224–30.
11. Wakabayashi Y, Yamada E, Yoshida T, et al. Arginine becomes an essential amino acid after massive resection of rat small intestine. J Biol Chem 1994;269: 32667–71.
12. Barbul A, Wasserkrug HL, Seifter E, et al. Immunostimulatory effects of arginine in normal and injured rats. J Surg Res 1980;29:228–35.
13. Ochoa JB, Udekwu AO, Billiar TR, et al. Nitrogen oxide levels in patients after trauma and during sepsis. Ann Surg 1991;214:621–6.
14. Tsuei BJ, Bernard AC, Barksdale AR, et al. Supplemental enteral arginine is metabolized to ornithine in injured patients. J Surg Res 2005;123:17–24.
15. Jacob TD, Ochoa JB, Udekwu AO, et al. Nitric oxide production is inhibited in trauma patients. J Trauma 1993;35:590–6 [discussion: 596–7].
16. Lovett JE III, Fink BF, Bernard A, et al. Analysis of nitric oxide activity in prevention of reperfusion injury. Ann Plast Surg 2001;46:269–73.
17. Ochoa JB, Strange J, Kearney P, et al. Effects of L-arginine on the proliferation of T lymphocyte subpopulations. JPEN J Parenter Enteral Nutr 2001;25:23–9.
18. Ochoa JB, Makarenkova V. T lymphocytes. Crit Care Med 2005;33:S510–3.
19. Zea AH, Rodriguez PC, Culotta KS, et al. L-arginine modulates CD3zeta expression and T cell function in activated human T lymphocytes. Cell Immunol 2004; 232:21–31.
20. Rodriguez PC, Zea AH, DeSalvo J, et al. L-arginine consumption by macrophages modulates the expression of CD3 zeta chain in T lymphocytes. J Immunol 2003;171:1232–9.
21. Taheri F, Ochoa JB, Faghiri Z, et al. L-arginine regulates the expression of the T cell receptor zeta chain (CD3zeta) in Jurkat cells. Clin Cancer Res 2001;7:958s–65.
22. Rodriguez PC, Ochoa AC. Arginine regulation by myeloid derived suppressor cells and tolerance in cancer: mechanisms and therapeutic perspectives. Immunol Rev 2008;222:180–91.
23. Ochoa AC, Zea AH, Hernandez C, et al. Arginase, prostaglandins, and myeloid-derived suppressor cells in renal cell carcinoma. Clin Cancer Res 2007;13: 721s–6.
24. Makarenkova VP, Bansal V, Matta BM, et al. CD11b+/Gr-1+ myeloid suppressor cells cause T cell dysfunction after traumatic stress. J Immunol 2006;176: 2085–94.

25. Gabrilovich DI, Bronte V, Chen SH, et al. The terminology issue for myeloid-derived suppressor cells. Cancer Res 2007;67:425.
26. Gabrilovich DI, Nagaraj S. Myeloid-derived suppressor cells as regulators of the immune system. Nat Rev Immunol 2009;9:162–74.
27. Bronte V, Serafini P, Apolloni E, et al. Tumor-induced immune dysfunctions caused by myeloid suppressor cells. J Immunother 2001;24:431–46.
28. Barksdale AR, Bernard AC, Maley ME, et al. Regulation of arginase expression by T helper II cytokines and isoproterenol. Surgery 2004;135:527–35.
29. Bernard AC, Fitzpatrick EA, Maley ME, et al. Beta adrenoceptor regulation of macrophage arginase activity. Surgery 2000;127(4):412–8.
30. Rodriguez PC, Hernandez CP, Quiceno D, et al. Arginase I in myeloid suppressor cells is induced by COX-2 in lung carcinoma. J Exp Med 2005;202:931–9.
31. Bansal V, Ochoa JB. Arginine availability, arginase, and the immune response. Curr Opin Clin Nutr Metab Care 2003;6:223–8.
32. Bansal V, Syres KM, Makarenkova V, et al. Interactions between fatty acids and arginine metabolism: implications for the design of immune-enhancing diets. JPEN J Parenter Enteral Nutr 2005;29:S75–80.
33. Okamoto Y, Okano K, Izuishi K, et al. Attenuation of the systemic inflammatory response and infectious complications after gastrectomy with preoperative oral arginine and omega-3 fatty acids supplemented immunonutrition. World J Surg 2009;33:1815–21.
34. Mirza N, Fishman M, Fricke I, et al. All-trans-retinoic acid improves differentiation of myeloid cells and immune response in cancer patients. Cancer Res 2006;66:9299–307.
35. Ochoa JB, Makarenkova V, Bansal V. A rational us of immune enhancing diets: when should we use dietary arginine supplementation? Nutr Clin Pract 2004;19(3):216–25.
36. Ochoa JB. Separating pharmaconutrition from classic nutrition goals: a necessary step. Crit Care Med 2008;36:347–8.
37. Braga M, Gianotti L, Radaelli G, et al. Perioperative immunonutrition in patients undergoing cancer surgery: results of a randomized double-blind phase 3 trial. Arch Surg 1999;134:428–33.
38. Braga M, Gianotti L, Vignali A, et al. Preoperative oral arginine and n-3 fatty acid supplementation improves the immunometabolic host response and outcome after colorectal resection for cancer. Surgery 2002;132:805–14.
39. Kudsk KA, Minard G, Croce MA, et al. A randomized trial of isonitrogenous enteral diets after severe trauma. An immune-enhancing diet reduces septic complications. Ann Surg 1996;224:531–40.

Fish Oil in Critical Illness: Mechanisms and Clinical Applications

Renee D. Stapleton, MD, MSc[a],*, Julie M. Martin, MS, RD, CD[b],
Konstantin Mayer, MD[c]

KEYWORDS

- Omega-3 fatty acids • Fish oil • Acute lung injury • Sepsis
- Critical illness • Mechanical ventilation

The omega-3 fatty acids (FAs) found in fish oil are essential and are thought to play a key role as both a preventative and a therapy for coronary artery disease, diabetes, hypertension, arthritis, cancer, and other inflammatory and autoimmune disorders.[1] In the last decade, research of omega-3 FAs has focused on their role in modulating the inflammatory response and, in turn, on their potential benefit in critically ill patients. Sepsis is the leading cause of death in critically ill patients in the United States[2] and causes most cases of acute lung injury (ALI), an inflammatory syndrome of hypoxemic respiratory failure and diffuse pulmonary infiltrates.[3] The physiologic manifestations of sepsis and other critical illnesses including ALI and trauma are believed to result from massive activation of the inflammatory cascade as well as immunosuppression or immunoparalysis.[4–6] One feature of uncontrolled activation of the inflammatory response involves excessive production of proinflammatory cytokines and lipid-derived inflammatory mediators termed eicosanoids.[7] As such, a relatively new area of research has investigated whether or not lipids administered during critical illness may modify the stress response, and thus, improve clinical outcomes.

This article examines mechanisms of action by which omega-3 FAs may affect inflammation. We also discuss clinical research to date in which omega-3 FAs have been are administered both enterally and parenterally. Although research conducted

[a] Division of Pulmonary and Critical Care, Department of Medicine, University of Vermont College of Medicine, 149 Beaumont Avenue, HSRF 222, Burlington, VT 05405, USA
[b] Division of Pulmonary and Critical Care, Department of Medicine, University of Vermont College of Medicine, 149 Beaumont Avenue, HSRF 230, Burlington, VT 05405, USA
[c] University of Giessen Lung Center (UGLC), Medical Clinic II, Justus-Liebig-University, Klinikstr 36, D-35392, Giessen, Germany
* Corresponding author.
E-mail address: renee.stapleton@uvm.edu

Crit Care Clin 26 (2010) 501–514
doi:10.1016/j.ccc.2010.04.009
0749-0704/10/$ – see front matter © 2010 Elsevier Inc. All rights reserved.
criticalcare.theclinics.com

in all critically ill patient populations is examined, more attention is focused on patients with sepsis or ALI due to their amplified inflammatory response.

OMEGA-3 FATTY ACIDS: MECHANISMS OF ACTION

Although a normal response to infection or injury, inflammation can occur on a massive and uncontrolled scale, thus leading to excessive tissue damage and potential worsening of illness. This overactivation of the inflammatory response is characterized by high levels of cytokines, including tumor necrosis factor (TNF)-α, interleukin (IL)-1β, and IL-6, which have been implicated in the pathologenesis of severe sepsis and ALI.[5,7]

The inflammatory response can be affected by phospholipids present in the membranes of immune cells including macrophages, monocytes, and neutrophils. The fatty acid composition of cell membranes influences membrane fluidity, which in turn can affect the activity of membrane-bound enzymes, receptors, transporters, and lipid-based second messenger systems (lipid signaling).[8–10] Additionally, particular FAs also affect the inflammatory response by altering the substrate for production of lipid inflammatory mediators including the eicosanoids. The primary unsaturated long-chain FAs in human cellular membranes include the omega-3 FAs eicosapentaenoic acid (EPA) and docosahexanoic acid (DHA), the omega-6 FA arachidonic acid (AA), and the omega-9 FA oleic acid.[11] Leukocyte membrane phospholipids usually are composed of approximately 30% polyunsaturated FAs (PUFAs).[11] Under a typical Western diet, most PUFAs are omega-6 FAs (primarily AA), while only a small percentage are omega-3 FAs.[12] AA is an omega-6 fatty acid formed from linoleic acid, which is present in high concentration in corn, sunflower, soybean, and safflower oils. With activation of the inflammatory cascade, macrophages are able to mobilize up to 40% of their membrane lipid content by phospolipases to produce free AA.[11] Free AA then is metabolized further by cycloxygenase (COX) and 5-lipoxygenase (LOX) into proinflammatory eicosanoids, including the 2-series thromboxanes and prostaglandins and the 4-series leukotrienes (Fig. 1).[11] The affects of these eicosanoids in inflammation are well understood, especially thromboxane A_2 (TXA_2), prostaglandin E_2 (PGE_2), and leukotriene B_4 (LTB_4).[13] TXA_2 increases platelet aggregation, leukocyte adhesion, vascular permeability, pulmonary vasoconstriction, and

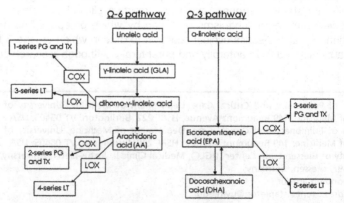

Fig. 1. Eicosanoids derived from Omega-6 and Omega-3 Fatty Acids. Abbreviations: AA, arachidonic acid; COX, cycloxygenase; DHA, docosahexanoic acid; EPA, eicosapentaenoic acid; LOX, lipoxygenase; LT, leukotriene; PG, prostaglandin; TX, thromboxane.

bronchoconstriction,[14,15] and it has prothrombotic effects that may lead to tissue ischemia.[11] PGE_2 induces vasodilation, fever, and vascular permeability during sepsis.[11,13,14] LTB_4 activates leukocytes, resulting in the generation of reactive oxygen species, release of proteases such as elastase, synthesis of lipid mediators, and neutrophil chemotaxis.[11] Of interest, platelet-activating factor (PAF) is tightly involved in the regulation of eicosanoid release through a two-step activation process including phospholipase A2-dependent cleavage of membrane phospholipids, resulting simultaneously in the release of the active lipid mediator and free AA.[16]

The omega-3 FAs EPA and DHA are essential for normal growth and development and are highly enriched in the cell membranes of the brain and the eye. They have several known anti-inflammatory mechanisms of action and are effective in the secondary prevention of myocardial infarction; they additionally may have a role in the prevention and treatment of diabetes, hypertension, hypertriglyceridemia, and cancer as well as autoimmune disorders.[1] The richest source of EPA and DHA is in fish oil, and increased dietary consumption increases incorporation into inflammatory cell membranes.[17] Omega-3 FAs replace AA in the phospholipid membrane; therefore, AA concentration is reduced, and production of the highly inflammatory AA-derived eicosanoids is decreased due to substrate restriction. In addition to this replacement mechanism, EPA also inhibits the metabolism of AA into the inflammatory eicosanoids and is itself metabolized to a far less inflammatory series of eicosanoids (PGE_3 and LTB_5) than those derived from AA.[18,19] Fish oil has been shown in animal studies to decrease production of AA-derived eicosanoid inflammatory mediators by 40% to 70%.[20,21] In murine models of ALI, endogenous synthesis of omega-3 fatty acids in transgenic mice[22] or intravenous infusion of a fish oil-based lipid emulsion decreased edema formation, leukocyte infiltration, and sickness behavior.[23,24] Exogenous delivery of fish oil reduced TNF-α, while endogenous synthesis of omega-3 FAs did not alter TNF-α generation but reduced generation of the proinflammatory nuclear factor (NF)-kappa B.

An additional mechanism of action involving EPA and DHA has also been described recently. It is now known that resolution of inflammation is an active process, rather than simply absence of inflammatory signals.[25] Novel molecules called resolvins, protectins, and maresins[26,27]—lipid mediators derived from EPA and DHA with potent pro-resolving, anti-inflammatory, and neuroprotective properties[28,29]—have been found to play an important role in the repair and resolution of inflammation.[30] Resolvin (Rv) E1 and Protectin D1 are quite well characterized resolving mediators effective in animal models of colitis and airway inflammation.[31–33] RvE1 has been found to activate cells by binding to an adopted orphan receptor called ChemR23, thereby decreasing the generation of the proinflammatory nuclear factor (NF)-kappa B.[34] In addition, it competes with binding of LTB4 to its receptor,[35] leading to decreased activation of leukocytes. Administration of resolvin D2 has been shown to improve outcomes in a murine model of abdominal sepsis.[36]

In addition to mechanisms at the level of the cell membrane and involving resolvins and protectins, omega-3 FAs also may have direct cardiac effects by interfering with ion channels in cardiac myocytes. It has been suggested that omega-3 FAs or derived metabolites may inhibit the delayed rectifier potassium channel or fast voltage-dependent sodium channels and L-type calcium channels, thereby reducing the arrhythmogenic potential in cardiac myocytes.[37] Of interest, one single-center study in cardiac surgical patients suggested a reduced occurrence of postoperative atrial fibrillation after oral administration of omega-3 FAs.[38] These data are supported by another single-center study in 102 cardiac surgical patients receiving either an intravenous fish oil-based lipid emulsion (Omegaven, Fresenius Kabi, Bad Homburg,

Germany) compared with a standard soybean-based lipid emulsion (Lipoven, Frese-nius Kabi, Bad Homburg, Germany). The authors reported reduced occurrence of post-operative atrial fibrillation and shorter length of stay in the intensive care unit (ICU) and hospital.[39]

In addition, omega-3 FAs may affect the autonomic nervous system and the neuro-endocrine axis. Prior studies have demonstrated that dietary EPA and DHA reduce resting heart rate and improve heart rate variability.[40,41] EPA and DHA also reduced the generation of adrenocorticotropic hormone and norepinephrine In volunteers challenged with intravenous endotoxin,[42,43] and a fish oil-containing lipid emulsion in postoperative critically ill patients resulted in a trend to lower body temperature in a single-center study.[44]

Although supplementation with omega-3 FAs generally is thought to reduce the unfavorable inflammatory effects of omega-6 FAs through the previously mentioned mechanisms,[45] there is also one omega-6 fatty acid, gamma-linolenic acid (GLA), that may provide benefit in critical illness. GLA is found in evening primrose oil, black current seeds, and borage oil, and it is rapidly converted to dihomo-GLA, which is incorporated into immune cell phospholipids and should theoretically be further metabolized to AA.[46] However, GLA actually reduces the availability of AA and synthesis of AA-derived eicosanoids through unclear mechanisms. Dihomo-GLA is further metabolized to prostaglandin E_1 (PGE_1), a strong pulmonary and systemic vasodilator (see **Fig. 1**).[47] In animal models of critical illness, GLA together with EPA and DHA have an additive effect to decrease inflammation and organ failure.[48] With this potential additive effect in mind, as will be discussed, much of the omega-3 research in critically ill patients with sepsis and ALI has been conducted using a commercially available enteral feeding formula that contains EPA, DHA, GLA, and several antioxidants.[49–51]

ENTERAL OMEGA-3 FAS IN CRITICAL ILLNESS

Commercially available enteral nutrition formulas with added fish oil have been studied in mixed ICU populations, separately in surgical or medical ICU patients, and in patients with trauma or burns. Interpretation of data in this area is difficult due to differing amounts of EPA and DHA present in various enteral formulations (1.0 to 6.6 g/L) and the inclusion of other micronutrients in the formulas.[52] Furthermore, the degree of clinical response to fish oil-containing formulas may vary between patients due to the type and severity of illnesses in the populations studied.

Three randomized clinical trials (RCTs) using a commercial feeding formula (Oxepa, Abbott Nutrition, Abbott Laboratories, Columbus, OH, USA) that contains EPA, DHA, GLA, and several antioxidants in critically ill patients have been completed and pub-lished (**Table 1**). Two of these RCTs included only patients with ALI,[49,50] and the third studied patients with sepsis[51] (although nearly all of the patients in the third RCT had single-organ lung failure, ie, ALI). All three of these trials randomized patients to receive either the enteral formula containing EPA, DHA, GLA, and antioxidants (Oxepa) or an isonitrogenous, high-fat, low-carbohydrate enteral feeding formula that did not contain fish oil. One of the studies used a different control formula that was equal in fat content (55% fat) but differed in lipid composition from the control formulation used by the other two studies.[51] In studies from Gadek and colleagues[49] and Singer and colleagues,[50] the lipid content of the control formula was 97% corn oil, which is high in linoleic acid, an omega-6 fatty acid. The lipid in the control formula in the study by Pontes-Arrudes and colleagues[51] was 55.8% canola oil, 14% corn oil, 20% medium chain triglycerides (MCT), 7% high oleic safflower oil, and 3.2% soy lecithin.

Table 1
Published randomized controlled trials comparing a commercial enteral feeding formula enriched with EPA, DHA, GLA, and antioxidants to another high-fat enteral feeding formula without fish oils

	Gadek et al[49]	Singer et al[50]	Pontes-Arruda et al[51]
Population studied	ARDS	ALI	Severe Sepsis
	n = 146	n = 100	n = 165
Study design	R, C, DB	R, C	R, C, DB
Mean fatty acid intake (g/d)			
EPA	6.9	5.4	4.9
DHA	2.9	2.5	2.2
GLA	5.8	5.1	4.6
Significant findings[a]			
Improved oxygenation	Yes	Yes[b]	Yes
Reduced ICU length of stay	Yes	No	Yes
Reduced ventilator time	Yes	Yes[c]	Yes
Reduced 28-day mortality	No	Yes	Yes
Fewer new organ failures	Yes	Not assessed	Yes

Abbreviations: ALI, acute lung injury; ARDS, acute respiratory distress syndrome; C, controlled; DB, double blind; DHA, docosahexaenoic acid; EPA, eicosapentaenoic acid; FA, fatty acid; GLA, gamma-linolenic acid; R, randomized.
 [a] Statistically significant ($P<0.05$).
 [b] Days 4, 7 only.
 [c] Day 7 only.

In the first study, subjects in the treatment group received approximately 7 g EPA, 3g DHA, and 6g GLA per day.[49] Serial bronchoalveolar lavage (BAL) was done at study entry, day 4, and day 7. The treatment group had improved oxygenation at days 4 and 7 ($P<.0499$), decreased duration of mechanical ventilation ($P = .027$), reduced BAL fluid neutrophil count (representing decreased lung inflammation) at day 4 ($P = .008$), decreased ICU length of stay ($P = .016$), and fewer new organ failures ($P = .018$). Mortality was 16% in the treatment group and 25% in the control group ($P = .165$).

In the second trial by Singer and colleagues, patients in the EPA/DHA/GLA/antioxidant group had a shorter, but statistically insignificant, duration of mechanical ventilation at day 14.[50] Hospital length of stay was not different between the two groups, but oxygenation was improved at days 4 and 7 ($P<.05$). Hospital mortality in this study was very high (>75%) in both groups 3 months after the intervention.

The third trial in patients with sepsis (most of whom had ALI) found significant increases in ICU-free days ($P<.001$), ventilator-free days ($P<.001$), and 28-day survival (52% versus 33%, $P = .04$) in the treatment group.[51] All patients tolerated near-goal enteral feeding. Development of new organ dysfunctions was also reduced ($P<.001$) in patients receiving the formula enriched with EPA, DHA, and GLA.

In a meta-analysis of these three studies, the use of the treatment formula enriched with EPA, DHA, GLA, and antioxidants was associated with a 60% reduction in the risk of 28-day all-cause mortality (odds ratio [OR] = 0.40; 95% confidence interval [CI] = 0.24 to 0.68; $P = .001$).[47] Significant reductions also were found in the risk of developing new organ failures (OR = 0.17; 95% CI = 0.08 to 0.34; $P<.0001$), time on mechanical ventilation (standardized mean difference [SMD] = 0.56; 95% CI = 0.32

to 0.79; $P<.0001$), and in length of stay in the ICU (SMD = 0.51; 95% CI = 0.27 to 0.74; $P<.0001$) in patients who received the formula containing fish oil. A second meta-analysis by Marik and Zaloga (that also included additional studies using enteral formulas containing other "immunomodulatory" nutrients) confirmed the findings reporting improved mortality (OR 0.42, CI 0.26 to 0.68, $P<.001$), secondary infections (OR 0.45, 95% CI 0.25 to 0.79, $P<.005$), and length of stay (weighted mean difference [WMD] -6.28 days, 95% CI -9.92 to -2.64) in patients who received enteral formulas that contained fish oil.[52] These studies also have been reviewed as part of the Canadian Clinical Practice Guidelines for enteral nutrition supplemented with fish oils, available at www.criticalcarenutrition.com, and they have been evaluated in the Society of Critical Care Medicine (SCCM) and American Society for Parenteral and Enteral Nutrition (A.S.P.E.N) 2009 Critical Care Guidelines.[53,54]

Two additional publications from the randomized clinical trial by Gadek and colleagues[49] investigated mechanisms of action of EPA, DHA, GLA and antioxidants in patients with ALI. The first investigation reported on the antioxidant status of the participants with ALI and compared them with a group of healthy controls.[55] At enrollment, the patients with ALI had reduced levels of antioxidant vitamins and were found to be in a state of oxidative stress (as measured by total radical antioxidant potential [TRAP] and lipid peroxide levels) compared with healthy controls. After receiving the treatment formula, the levels of oxidative stress were not significantly reduced, but plasma levels of β-carotene and α-tocopherol were restored to normal, while lipid peroxide levels did not increase, thus suggesting the antioxidants may have protected against further lipid peroxidation. The second ancillary study reported a significantly reduced level of IL-8 (a potent inflammatory cytokine and neutrophil chemoattractant) in BAL fluid of patients in the treatment group ($P = .05$), as well as a trend toward reduced levels of IL-6, LTB_4 and TNF-α.[56] Because the previously mentioned trials investigated a single enteral formula (Oxepa) containing multiple pharmaconutrients, the benefit attributed exclusively to omega-3 FAs is unknown.

Other enteral nutritional formulas enriched with omega-3 FAs have been studied in critically ill patients suffering from trauma, surgery, or burns. These formulas usually are supplemented with additional nutrients thought to affect immune function, such as the amino acids arginine or glutamine or antioxidant vitamins.[57] The previously mentioned meta-analysis by Marik and Zaloga analyzed data from enteral nutrition studies and separated the studies by the types of micronutrients included in the formula (fish oil, arginine, or glutamine) and the population studied (surgical ICU, medical ICU, mixed ICU, burns, or trauma).[52] All studies in nonmedical ICU patients included in this meta-analysis used a formula that also contained arginine. Mixed ICU patients with sepsis and ALI improved with the addition of fish oil to enteral feedings, but supplementation with fish oil and arginine (with or without glutamine) did not show benefit for patients in the surgical ICU or for those with trauma or burns.[52] Another meta-analysis has suggested that formulas containing arginine may benefit elective surgical patients but may be harmful to critically ill patients with sepsis.[58] Use of arginine-containing formulas in critically ill patients showed a trend toward higher mortality, while there was no such effect in elective surgical patients.[58] Therefore, a negative effect or lack of benefit with use of these formulas that contain both arginine and fish oil in critically ill patients may be related to the arginine and not the omega-3 FAs, especially in critically ill medical ICU patients with sepsis.

When pharmaconutrients are combined with macronutrients in enteral feedings, it is difficult to generalize study results. Two recently completed but not yet published RCTs of omega-3 FAs in patients with ALI were designed to dissociate the pharmaconutrients from enteral feedings; the pharmaconutrients were administered enterally as medications while patients received standard enteral nutrition regimens per their treating physicians.[59,60] The preliminary results of these two recent RCTs were presented orally at the American Thoracic Society (ATS) International Conference held May 15 to 20, 2009, in San Diego, California. Both of these trials appear to challenge the positive results found in the previous RCTs using the enteral formula containing EPA, DHA, GLA, and antioxidants.[59,60] The first trial, the OMEGA study, is a large phase 3 RCT conducted by the National Institutes of Health, National Heart Lung and Blood Institute Acute Respiratory Distress Syndrome Network (ARDSnet) to investigate whether an enteral supplement (delivered twice daily) containing EPA, DHA, GLA, and antioxidants would have benefit in patients with ALI.[60] This RCT was stopped due to futility in March 2009 after accrual of 272 of the planned 1000 patients. The enteral supplement did not improve the outcomes of ventilator-free days at day 28, ICU-free days at day 28, or death at 60 days. The second study by Stapleton and colleagues[59] reported at the conference was a phase 2 randomized, double-blind, placebo-controlled trial of enteral fish oil (EPA and DHA) in 90 critically ill patients with ALI. Fish oil or a saline placebo was given enterally as a medication, separate from enteral or parenteral nutrition in this trial. The primary endpoint was BAL fluid IL-8, and secondary endpoints included clinical outcomes as well as biomarkers of inflammation and injury, oxygenation, and lung compliance. None of the primary or secondary endpoints were significantly different between the treatment and control groups. Based on the preliminary results available from these two studies, the effect of enteral fish oil supplementation in patients with ALI and sepsis is unclear. One limitation of the three earlier studies using the enteral formula enriched with EPA, DHA, GLA, and antioxidants in patients with ALI is the use of a control formula in two of the studies[49,50] that was high in linoleic acid, an omega-6 fatty acid. It is unclear why the promising effect of the previous studies could not be reproduced in the two newer studies.[59,60] There are differences between the designs of the different studies including the intervention, control formulas, and continuous administration versus bolus administration of the agent.

Most studies investigating the effects of enteral fish oils included in an enteral feeding formula with other nutrients including arginine, glutamine, or antioxidants have been in nonmedical ICU patents with trauma,[61,62] burns,[63,64] or surgery[65,66] and they have found no benefits in mortality, length of hospital stay, or rates of new infections. Many of these studies were small, however, with some intending only to detect differences in biochemical parameters or biomarkers. One large multicenter study in septic patients examined the effect of fish oil, arginine, and nucleotides and did demonstrate an improvement in mortality.[67] In subgroup analysis, however, the overall effect was largely due to patients with a low Acute Physiologic and Health Evaluation Score (APACHE II), and mortality was actually worse in patients with a APACHE II score greater than 25. Therefore the effect of enteral fish oil in these populations is not clear. This conclusion, however, is based on a small number of studies in each population.[52] Additional research is needed before any definitive recommendations can be made about enteral omega-3 fatty acid supplementation in critically ill patients.

INCLUSION OF OMEGA-3 FAS IN PARENTERAL NUTRITION

As with enteral delivery, the specific type of FAs in lipid emulsions administered parenterally may also impact the inflammatory response in critical illness. Soybean oil, consisting of roughly 54% linoleic acid (an omega-6 fatty acid), is the lipid traditionally used in parenteral nutrition (PN).[68] Concern has been raised over the potential proinflammatory, procoagulatory, and immunosuppressive properties of linoleic acid. However, clinical trials using these emulsions have provided conflicting evidence.[69]

A meta-analysis of two studies[70,71] where standard lipids in PN were compared with no lipids suggested that PN with standard lipids may result in a higher infectious complication rate ($P = .02$) than PN without lipids, although mortality was not different between the two groups.[72] This concern about lipid emulsions has led to new formulations that partially replace soybean oil with other oils including MCT, olive oil, or fish oil.[69]

Human studies of parenteral fish oil emulsions have been conducted. In a study by Mayer and colleagues,[73] 21 patients who required PN due to intolerance of enteral nutrition were randomized in an open-label trial to receive an omega-3 fatty acid lipid emulsion (Omegaven; Fresenius Kabi, Bad Homburg, Germany) or a standard omega-6 lipid emulsion (Lipoven; Fresenius Kabi) for 5 days. The omega-3 rich emulsion increased plasma concentrations of omega-3 free FAs and reversed the omega-3/omega-6 ratio toward favoring EPA and DHA over AA, reaching maximum effect in 3 days. In patients receiving the fish oil emulsion, EPA and DHA rapidly incorporated into mononuclear leukocyte cell membranes, increasing threefold in concentration. Ex vivo, these cells produced 30% less TNF-α, IL 1-β, IL-6, IL-8, and IL-10 when stimulated by endotoxin. However, serum cytokine levels between the patients receiving parenteral omega-3 FAs and the standard lipid emulsion were not different. In another study by the same authors, 10 patients with septic shock requiring PN were randomized to receive fish oil fortified Omegaven or the standard omega-6 rich Lipoven for 10 days.[74] C-reactive protein levels and leukocyte counts decreased in patients receiving the omega-3 emulsion and increased in patients receiving the omega-6 emulsion, with a trend toward significance ($P = .08$ and $P = .09$, respectively). Patients in the omega-6 group trended toward longer ventilation time ($P = .07$). LTB_5 increased in the fish oil group, approaching an LTB_4/LTB_5 ratio of almost 20% by the end of the study infusion period. These results support the hypothesis that parenteral omega-3 FAs in patients with septic shock modulate inflammatory mediator production and attenuate inflammation.

In a prospective, open-label trial, infusion of omega-3 FAs during PN (Omegaven) improved diagnosis-related clinical outcomes in critically ill patients with major abdominal surgery (n = 255), peritonitis and abdominal sepsis (n = 276), nonabdominal sepsis (n = 16), multitrauma (n = 59), severe head injury (n = 18), or other diagnoses (n = 37).[75] Both ICU and hospital lengths of stay were reduced significantly (both $P<.001$) with doses of greater than 0.05 g fish oil/kg/d, and patients receiving greater than 0.15 g/kg/d needed less antibiotic treatment. Mortality was significantly decreased ($P<.05$) in patients receiving greater than 0.10 g fish oil/kg/d. In an analysis of patients by diagnosis, according to mean fish oil dose received, patients with severe head injury ($P<.0001$), multiple trauma ($P<.0001$), and abdominal sepsis ($P = .0027$), had significantly lower mortality. These results suggest benefit from parenteral omega-3, but this study was not controlled or blinded. Another recent trial randomized patients with severe acute pancreatitis to receive either a combination of 20% Omegaven plus 80% Lipoven or Lipoven alone.[76] There were no significant differences in white blood cell count, C-reactive protein, rates of organ dysfunction, infectious complications, or ICU length of stay. However, IL-6 decreased to a significantly greater degree between baseline and day 6 in patients in the fish oil group ($P<.05$). Additionally, oxygenation was significantly increased ($P<.05$), and there was a significantly decreased need for renal replacement therapy ($P<.05$) in the patients receiving fish oil.

In contrast to the positive results of the previous studies, which were largely in surgically critically ill patients, a randomized, double-blind, controlled trial in critically ill medical patients found no clear medical benefit to parenteral omega-3 FAs.[77] In that study, 166 medical ICU patients were randomized to receive a mixture of medium- and long-chain triglycerides (Lipofundin MCT; Braun Medical, Melsungen, Germany) or a combination of Omegaven and Lipofundin MCT for 7 days. Based on data from a prior study,[78] this RCT was designed to detect a biologic endpoint: more rapid reduction in IL-6 and greater monocyte expression of HLA-DR, a marker of immune competence, in the omega-3 group. The authors found no differences in IL-6 or HLA-DR between the treatment groups, nor did they detect differences in mortality, duration of mechanical ventilation, ICU length of stay, infectious complications, other inflammatory markers, or bleeding events.[77] One possible explanation for this lack of effect is that the start of the study occurred after the initial inflammatory process was already resolving. In addition, the study may have been underpowered. This study also used a control lipid emulsion that was lower in omega-6 FAs (due to the presence of MCT) than most standard lipid emulsions, and thus may have been less inflammatory.[77] Recently, another single-center study in patients with the systemic inflammatory response syndrome was published where a parenteral lipid emulsion of MCT, soybean oil, and fish oil was compared with a lipid emulsion of MCT and soybean oil alone (Lipofundin-MCT).[79] The authors reported a faster reduction in IL-6, improved ventilation parameters, and a trend toward reduced hospital length of stay ($P<.079$).

No adverse effects have been reported with the administration of lipid emulsions fortified with fish oil, suggesting it is safe in critically ill patients.[69] Because available research provides conflicting data on the effects of parenteral omega-3 FAs in critically ill patients, its influence on inflammatory processes and clinical outcomes remains unclear.

SUMMARY

Although much is known about the mechanism of action of omega-3 FAs and their effect on cytokines and inflammatory mediators from research with animals, their effects on clinical outcomes in critically ill patients are not entirely clear, and further research is needed to determine any benefit. Trials of nutritional support and micronutrients, including omega-3 FAs, in critically ill patients are especially difficult to conduct and interpret for multiple reasons. First, patient enrollment can be difficult because of issues with surrogate consent and the short enrollment periods in most studies (eg, most trial require enrollment within 24 to 48 hours after ICU admission in an effort to initiate the agents early in the course of critical illness). Second, critically ill patients are a very heterogeneous population and present with a wide variety of severe medical illnesses. This heterogeneity means that large numbers of patients are required to demonstrate an effect.[80] Third, the delivery of nutrition and micronutrients is frequently interrupted or poorly tolerated in ICU patients, thus resulting in decreased delivery of the agent being studied, especially if it is enteral. Fourth, in many studies of enteral and parenteral nutrients, many agents frequently are combined into one formula, and therefore the effect produced by a single agent cannot be determined. Fifth, choice of control group agent in many trials is also in issue. Finally, dosing data on both enteral and parenteral omega-3 FAs in critically ill patients are very sparse.

Prior research demonstrating positive effects of enteral omega-3 FAs in patients with sepsis and ALI involved the continuous administration of one enteral formula fortified with EPA, DHA, GLA, and antioxidants.[49–51] These data are challenged by the use of bolus omega-3 FAs, either as a single enteral agent[59] or as part of an enteral immune-modulating cocktail.[60] Studies of parenteral omega-3 FAs suggesting a benefit have been conducted using a particular lipid emulsion (Omegaven) and are not yet conclusive.[73–77] After understanding the limitations of all the previous studies and gaining insight into possible dosing-, timing-, and application-dependent effects, it is clear that additional randomized, double-blinded, controlled trials in which omega-3 FAs are administered separately from feedings (and the feeding formulas are devoid of other micronutrients) and the control agent is an inert placebo are needed to definitively inform patient care.

REFERENCES

1. Simopoulos AP. Essential fatty acids in health and chronic disease. Am J Clin Nutr 1999;70(Suppl 3):560S–9S.
2. Angus DC, Linde-Zwirble WT, Lidicker J, et al. Epidemiology of severe sepsis in the United States: analysis of incidence, outcome, and associated costs of care. Crit Care Med 2001;29(7):1303–10.
3. Wheeler AP, Bernard GR. Acute lung injury and the acute respiratory distress syndrome: a clinical review. Lancet 2007;369(9572):1553–64.
4. Cohen J. The immunopathogenesis of sepsis. Nature 2002;420(6917):885–91.
5. Hotchkiss RS, Karl IE. The pathophysiology and treatment of sepsis. N Engl J Med 2003;348(2):138–50.
6. Volk HD, Reinke P, Docke WD. Clinical aspects: from systemic inflammation to immunoparalysis. Chem Immunol 2000;74:162–77.
7. Calder PC. N-3 polyunsaturated fatty acids and inflammation: from molecular biology to the clinic. Lipids 2003;38(4):343–52.
8. Stubbs CD, Smith AD. The modification of mammalian membrane polyunsaturated fatty acid composition in relation to membrane fluidity and function. Biochim Biophys Acta 1984;779(1):89–137.
9. Murphy MG. Dietary fatty acids and membrane protein function. J Nutr Biochem 1990;1(2):68–79.
10. Calder PC. The relationship between the fatty acid composition of immune cells and their function. Prostaglandins Leukot Essent Fatty Acids 2008;79(3–5):101–8.
11. Bulger EM, Maier RV. Lipid mediators in the pathophysiology of critical illness. Crit Care Med 2000;28(Suppl 4):N27–36.
12. Palombo JD, Lydon EE, Chen PL, et al. Fatty acid composition of lung, macrophage, and surfactant phospholipids after short-term enteral feeding with n-3 lipids. Lipids 1994;29(9):643–9.
13. Tilley SL, Coffman TM, Koller BH. Mixed messages: modulation of inflammation and immune responses by prostaglandins and thromboxanes. J Clin Invest 2001;108(1):15–23.
14. Harris SG, Padilla J, Koumas L, et al. Prostaglandins as modulators of immunity. Trends Immunol 2002;23(3):144–50.
15. Petrak RA, Balk RA, Bone RC. Prostaglandins, cyclo-oxygenase inhibitors, and thromboxane synthetase inhibitors in the pathogenesis of multiple systems organ failure. Crit Care Clin 1989;5(2):303–14.
16. Prescott SM, Zimmerman GA, McIntyre TM. Platelet-activating factor. J Biol Chem 1990;265(29):17381–4.
17. Marangoni F, Angeli MT, Colli S, et al. Changes of n-3 and n-6 fatty acids in plasma and circulating cells of normal subjects, after prolonged administration of 20:5 (EPA) and 22:6 (DHA) ethyl esters and prolonged washout. Biochim Biophys Acta 1993;1210(1):55–62.
18. Lee TH, Menica-Huerta JM, Shih C, et al. Characterization and biologic properties of 5,12-dihydroxy derivatives of eicosapentaenoic acid, including leukotriene B5 and the double lipoxygenase product. J Biol Chem 1984;259(4):2383–9.

19. Golman DW, Goetzl EJ. Human neutrophil chemotactic and degranulating activites of leukotriene B5 (LTB5) derived from eicosapentaenoic acid. Biochem Biophys Res Commun 1983;117:282–8.
20. Lee TH, Hoover RL, Williams JD, et al. Effect of dietary enrichment with eicosapentaenoic and docosahexaenoic acids on in vitro neutrophil and monocyte leukotriene generation and neutrophil function. N Engl J Med 1985;312(19):1217–24.
21. Whelan J, Broughton KS, Kinsella JE. The comparative effects of dietary alphalinolenic acid and fish oil on 4- and 5-series leukotriene formation in vivo. Lipids 1991;26(2):119–26.
22. Kang JX, Wang J, Wu L, et al. Transgenic mice: fat-1 mice convert n-6 to n-3 fatty acids. Nature 2004;427(6974):504.
23. Schaefer MB, Ott J, Mohr A, et al. Immunomodulation by n-3- versus n-6-rich lipid emulsions in murine acute lung injury–role of platelet-activating factor receptor. Crit Care Med 2007;35(2):544–54.
24. Mayer K, Kiessling A, Ott J, et al. Acute lung injury is reduced in fat-1 mice endogenously synthesizing n-3 fatty acids. Am J Respir Crit Care Med 2009; 179(6):474–83.
25. Ariel A, Serhan CN. Resolvins and protectins in the termination program of acute inflammation. Trends Immunol 2007;28(4):176–83.
26. Serhan CN, Yang R, Martinod K, et al. Maresins: novel macrophage mediators with potent antiinflammatory and proresolving actions. J Exp Med 2009;206(1): 15–23.
27. Serhan CN. Systems approach to inflammation resolution: identification of novel anti-inflammatory and proresolving mediators. J Thromb Haemost 2009;7(Suppl 1):44–8.
28. Serhan CN, Clish CB, Brannon J, et al. Novel functional sets of lipid-derived mediators with antiinflammatory actions generated from omega-3 fatty acids via cyclooxygenase 2-nonsteroidal antiinflammatory drugs and transcellular processing. J Exp Med 2000;192(8):1197–204.
29. Serhan CN, Hong S, Gronert K, et al. Resolvins: a family of bioactive products of omega-3 fatty acid transformation circuits initiated by aspirin treatment that counter proinflammation signals. J Exp Med 2002;196(8):1025–37.
30. Serhan CN, Chiang N, Van Dyke TE. Resolving inflammation: dual anti-inflammatory and proresolution lipid mediators. Nat Rev Immunol 2008;8(5):349–61.
31. Levy BD, Kohli P, Gotlinger K, et al. Protectin D1 is generated in asthma and dampens airway inflammation and hyperresponsiveness. J Immunol 2007; 178(1):496–502.
32. Haworth O, Cernadas M, Yang R, et al. Resolvin E1 regulates interleukin 23, interferon-gamma and lipoxin A4 to promote the resolution of allergic airway inflammation. Nat Immunol 2008;9(8):873–9.
33. Arita M, Yoshida M, Hong S, et al. Resolvin E1, an endogenous lipid mediator derived from omega-3 eicosapentaenoic acid, protects against 2,4,6-trinitrobenzene sulfonic acid-induced colitis. Proc Natl Acad Sci U S A 2005;102(21):7671–6.
34. Arita M, Bianchini F, Aliberti J, et al. Stereochemical assignment, anti-inflammatory properties, and receptor for the omega-3 lipid mediator resolvin E1. J Exp Med 2005;201(5):713–22.
35. Arita M, Ohira T, Sun YP, et al. Resolvin E1 selectively interacts with leukotriene B4 receptor BLT1 and ChemR23 to regulate inflammation. J Immunol 2007;178(6): 3912–7.
36. Spite M, Norling LV, Summers L, et al. Resolvin D2 is a potent regulator of leukocytes and controls microbial sepsis. Nature 2009;461(7268):1287–91.

37. Anand RG, Alkadri M, Lavie CJ, et al. The role of fish oil in arrhythmia prevention. J Cardiopulm Rehabil Prev 2008;28(2):92–8.
38. Calo L, Bianconi L, Colivicchi F, et al. N-3 Fatty acids for the prevention of atrial fibrillation after coronary artery bypass surgery: a randomized, controlled trial. J Am Coll Cardiol 2005;45(10):1723–8.
39. Heidt MC, Vician M, Stracke SK, et al. Beneficial effects of intravenously administered N-3 fatty acids for the prevention of atrial fibrillation after coronary artery bypass surgery: a prospective randomized study. Thorac Cardiovasc Surg 2009; 57(5):276–80.
40. O'Keefe JH Jr, Abuissa H, Sastre A, et al. Effects of omega-3 fatty acids on resting heart rate, heart rate recovery after exercise, and heart rate variability in men with healed myocardial infarctions and depressed ejection fractions. Am J Cardiol 2006;97(8):1127–30.
41. Geelen A, Brouwer IA, Schouten EG, et al. Effects of n-3 fatty acids from fish on premature ventricular complexes and heart rate in humans. Am J Clin Nutr 2005; 81(2):416–20.
42. Pluess TT, Hayoz D, Berger MM, et al. Intravenous fish oil blunts the physiological response to endotoxin in healthy subjects. Intensive Care Med 2007;33(5):789–97.
43. Michaeli B, Berger MM, Revelly JP, et al. Effects of fish oil on the neuro-endocrine responses to an endotoxin challenge in healthy volunteers. Clin Nutr 2007;26(1):70–7.
44. Berger MM, Tappy L, Revelly JP, et al. Fish oil after abdominal aorta aneurysm surgery. Eur J Clin Nutr 2008;62(9):1116–22.
45. Mayer K, Seeger W. Fish oil in critical illness. Curr Opin Clin Nutr Metab Care 2008;11(2):121–7.
46. Singer P, Shapiro H. Enteral omega-3 in acute respiratory distress syndrome. Curr Opin Clin Nutr Metab Care 2009;12(2):123–8.
47. Pontes-Arruda A, Demichele S, Seth A, et al. The use of an inflammation-modulating diet in patients with acute lung injury or acute respiratory distress syndrome: a meta-analysis of outcome data. JPEN J Parenter Enteral Nutr 2008;32(6):596–605.
48. Mancuso P, Whelan J, DeMichele SJ, et al. Dietary fish oil and fish and borage oil suppress intrapulmonary proinflammatory eicosanoid biosynthesis and attenuate pulmonary neutrophil accumulation in endotoxic rats. Crit Care Med 1997;25(7): 1198–206.
49. Gadek JE, DeMichele SJ, Karlstad MD, et al. Effect of enteral feeding with eicosapentaenoic acid, gamma-linolenic acid, and antioxidants in patients with acute respiratory distress syndrome. Enteral Nutrition in ARDS Study Group. Crit Care Med 1999;27(8):1409–20.
50. Singer P, Theilla M, Fisher H, et al. Benefit of an enteral diet enriched with eicosapentaenoic acid and gamma-linolenic acid in ventilated patients with acute lung injury. Crit Care Med 2006;34(4):1033–8.
51. Pontes-Arruda A, Aragao AM, Albuquerque JD. Effects of enteral feeding with eicosapentaenoic acid, gamma-linolenic acid, and antioxidants in mechanically ventilated patients with severe sepsis and septic shock. Crit Care Med 2006; 34(9):2325–33.
52. Marik PE, Zaloga GP. Immunonutrition in critically ill patients: a systematic review and analysis of the literature. Intensive Care Med 2008;34(11):1980–90.
53. Heyland DK. Nutrition clinical practice guidelines 4.1(b) composition of enteral nutrition: fish oils. Available at: http://www.criticalcarenutrition.com/docs/cpg/4.1bfish%20oils_FINAL.pdf. Accessed January 31, 2009.

54. McClave SA, Martindale RG, Vanek VW, et al. Guidelines for the provision and assessment of nutrition support therapy in the adult critically ill patient: Society of Critical Care Medicine (SCCM) and American Society for Parenteral and Enteral Nutrition (A.S.P.E.N). JPEN J Parenter Enteral Nutr 2009;33(3): 277–316.

55. Nelson JL, DeMichele SJ, Pacht ER, et al. Effect of enteral feeding with eicosapentaenoic acid, gamma-linolenic acid, and antioxidants on antioxidant status in patients with acute respiratory distress syndrome. JPEN J Parenter Enteral Nutr 2003;27(2):98–104.

56. Pacht ER, DeMichele SJ, Nelson JL, et al. Enteral nutrition with eicosapentaenoic acid, gamma-linolenic acid, and antioxidants reduces alveolar inflammatory mediators and protein influx in patients with acute respiratory distress syndrome. Crit Care Med 2003;31(2):491–500.

57. Calder PC. Immunonutrition in surgical and critically ill patients. Br J Nutr 2007; 98(Suppl 1):S133–9.

58. Heyland DK, Novak F, Drover JW, et al. Should immunonutrition become routine in critically ill patients? A systematic review of the evidence. JAMA 2001;286(8):944–53.

59. Stapleton RD, Martin TR, Gundel SJ, et al. A phase II, randomized, double-blind, placebo-controlled trial of fish oil (eicosapentaenoic acid and docosahexaenoic acid) on lung and systemic inflammation in patients with acute lung injury. Am J Respir Crit Care Med 2009;179:A2169.

60. Rice T. Trial of omega-3 fatty acid, gamma-linolenic acid and antioxidant supplemention in the management of acute lung injury (Omega). Presented at American Thoracic Society International Conference. San Diego (CA). May 2009;17.

61. Engel JM, Menges T, Neuhauser C, et al. [Effects of various feeding regimens in multiple trauma patients on septic complications and immune parameters]. Anasthesiol Intensivmed Notfallmed Schmerzther 1997;32(4):234–9 [in German].

62. Weimann A, Bastian L, Bischoff WE, et al. Influence of arginine, omega-3 fatty acids and nucleotide-supplemented enteral support on systemic inflammatory response syndrome and multiple organ failure in patients after severe trauma. Nutrition 1998;14(2):165–72.

63. Saffle JR, Wiebke G, Jennings K, et al. Randomized trial of immune-enhancing enteral nutrition in burn patients. J Trauma 1997;42(5):793–800 [discussion: 800–2].

64. Wibbenmeyer LA, Mitchell MA, Newel IM, et al. Effect of a fish oil and arginine-fortified diet in thermally injured patients. J Burn Care Res 2006; 27(5):694–702.

65. Cerra FB, Lehman S, Konstantinides N, et al. Effect of enteral nutrient on in vitro tests of immune function in ICU patients: a preliminary report. Nutrition 1990;6(1): 84–7 [discussion: 96–8].

66. Bower RH, Cerra FB, Bershadsky B, et al. Early enteral administration of a formula (Impact) supplemented with arginine, nucleotides, and fish oil in intensive care unit patients: results of a multicenter, prospective, randomized, clinical trial. Crit Care Med 1995;23(3):436–49.

67. Galban C, Montejo JC, Mesejo A, et al. An immune-enhancing enteral diet reduces mortality rate and episodes of bacteremia in septic intensive care unit patients. Crit Care Med 2000;28(3):643–8.

68. Suchner U, Katz DP, Furst P, et al. Impact of sepsis, lung injury, and the role of lipid infusion on circulating prostacyclin and thromboxane A(2). Intensive Care Med 2002;28(2):122–9.

69. Calder PC. Rationale for using new lipid emulsions in parenteral nutrition and a review of the trials performed in adults. Proc Nutr Soc 2009;68:252–60.

70. McCowen KC, Friel C, Sternberg J, et al. Hypocaloric total parenteral nutrition: effectiveness in prevention of hyperglycemia and infectious complications– a randomized clinical trial. Crit Care Med 2000;28(11):3606–11.
71. Battistella FD, Widergren JT, Anderson JT, et al. A prospective, randomized trial of intravenous fat emulsion administration in trauma victims requiring total parenteral nutrition. J Trauma 1997;43(1):52–8 [discussion: 58–60].
72. Heyland DK, Dhaliwal R, Drover JW, et al. Canadian clinical practice guidelines for nutrition support in mechanically ventilated, critically ill adult patients. JPEN J Parenter Enteral Nutr 2003;27(5):355–73.
73. Mayer K, Gokorsch S, Fegbeutel C, et al. Parenteral nutrition with fish oil modulates cytokine response in patients with sepsis. Am J Respir Crit Care Med 2003; 167(10):1321–8.
74. Mayer K, Fegbeutel C, Hattar K, et al. Omega-3 vs. omega-6 lipid emulsions exert differential influence on neutrophils in septic shock patients: impact on plasma fatty acids and lipid mediator generation. Intensive Care Med 2003;29(9): 1472–81.
75. Heller AR, Rossler S, Litz RJ, et al. Omega-3 fatty acids improve the diagnosis-related clinical outcome. Crit Care Med 2006;34(4):972–9.
76. Wang X, Li W, Li N, et al. Omega-3 fatty acids-supplemented parenteral nutrition decreases hyperinflammatory response and attenuates systemic disease sequelae in severe acute pancreatitis: a randomized and controlled study. JPEN J Parenter Enteral Nutr 2008;32(3):236–41.
77. Friesecke S, Lotze C, Kohler J, et al. Fish oil supplementation in the parenteral nutrition of critically ill medical patients: a randomised controlled trial. Intensive Care Med 2008;34(8):1411–20.
78. Weiss G, Meyer F, Matthies B, et al. Immunomodulation by perioperative administration of n-3 fatty acids. Br J Nutr 2002;87(Suppl 1):S89–94.
79. Barbosa VM, Miles EA, Calhau C, et al. Effects of a fish oil containing lipid emulsion on plasma phospholipid fatty acids, inflammatory markers, and clinical outcomes in septic patients: a randomized, controlled clinical trial. Crit Care 2010;14(1):R5.
80. Preiser JC, Chiolero R, Wernerman J. Nutritional papers in ICU patients: what lies between the lines? Intensive Care Med 2003;29(2):156–66.

Glutamine in Critical Illness: The Time Has Come, The Time Is Now

Lindsay-Rae B. Weitzel, PhD[a],*, Paul E. Wischmeyer, MD[b]

KEYWORDS

- Intensive Care • Glutamine • MODS
- Sepsis • Heat shock protein • Nutrition

Severe sepsis is now responsible for as much mortality as acute myocardial infarction in the United States (National Center for Health Statistics). An annualized increase in hospital sepsis incidence rates of 8.7% occurred from 164,000 cases in 1979 to approximately 660,000 cases in 2000.[1] The total percentage of hospital deaths due to sepsis has increased to 90% in the past 20 years.[2] The rate of severe sepsis continues to rise as does the number of people it kills. The percentage of severe sepsis cases among all sepsis cases increased continuously from 25.6% in 1993 to 43.8% in 2003 ($P<.001$). The age-adjusted rate of hospitalization for severe sepsis grew from 66.8 (± 0.16) to 132 (± 0.21) per 100,000 population ($P<.001$). The age-adjusted, population-based mortality rate for this same time period increased from 30.3 (± 0.11) to 49.7 (± 0.13) per 100,000 ($P<.001$).[3] Sepsis and inflammation commonly lead to multiple organ dysfunction syndrome (MODS), often the ultimate cause of death in an intensive care unit (ICU).[4] Sepsis-induced organ dysfunction, such as MODS, is thought associated with inflammation and a failure of cellular and tissue metabolism.[5] There are currently limited therapeutic options available to prevent MODS and mortality after onset of sepsis. One promising candidate for future sepsis and critical care therapeutics is using the body's innate stress substrates as

This work supported by National Institutes of Health Grants NCRR-K23 RR018379, NIDDK-RO3 DK073035, NIDDK-U01 DK069322, and NIGMS-RO1 GM078312—all to Paul E. Wischmeyer, MD.

[a] Department of Anesthesiology, Translational Pharmaconutrition (TPN) Research Laboratories, University of Colorado Denver, Research Complex 2, Box 8602, 12700 East 19th Avenue, Aurora, CO 80045, USA

[b] Department of Anesthesiology, Clinical and Translational Research, University of Colorado at Denver School of Medicine, Research Complex 2, Box 8602, 12700 East 19th Avenue, Aurora, CO 80045, USA

* Corresponding author.
E-mail address: Lindsay.Weitzel@ucdenver.edu

Crit Care Clin 26 (2010) 515–525
doi:10.1016/j.ccc.2010.04.006

pharmaconutrient interventions to induce endogenous protective pathways, such as the heat shock protein (HSP) response. Preservation or induction of these vital stress response pathways via substrates, such as glutamine (GLN), may be able to prevent MODS and, ultimately, mortality in ICU patients. The purpose of this review is to demonstrate how the well-established, low-risk, low-cost intervention of GLN therapy may protect organs against injury, attenuate inflammation, preserve metabolic function, and ultimately improve outcome in critically ill patients.

As is true with many amino acids, GLN metabolism is increased in those who are critically ill. In catabolic states, large amounts of GLN are released from muscle tissue[6] in what seems to be part of the fundamental evolutionarily conserved response to stress. Previous explanations for the release of GLN in periods of stress include its use as a fuel source for rapidly dividing cells, its use as a precursor for synthesis of nucleic acids, and its role in renal acid buffering.[7,8] Despite this massive release of GLN from muscle, it is well described in the literature that GLN levels are significantly decreased in critical illness and that this decrease is associated with an increase in mortality in critically ill patients.[9,10] This indicates that humans as a species have only evolved approximately 24 to 48 hours' worth of GLN stores to maintain GLN levels after injury.

Although GLN is classified as a nonessential amino acid and is synthesized de novo, it is commonly described as a conditionally essential amino acid, particularly in catabolic states.[11] Furthermore, recent data have revealed that after illness and injury GLN plays a vital role in inducing cellular protection pathways, modulation of the inflammatory response, and prevention of organ injury[10] Recently, an editorial proposed four main hypotheses through which GLN exerts its protective effects in critical illness while simultaneously indicating that further research is needed to elucidate specific mechanisms. These mechanisms include improved tissue protection, immune regulation, preservation of glutathione and antioxidant capacity, and preservation of cellular metabolism post injury.[12] Furthermore, new data indicate that GLN activates intracellular signaling pathways and regulates the expression of genes related to signal transduction, apoptosis, and metabolism.[13] These data support the hypothesis that release of GLN from muscle acts as a stress signal to the organism to turn on genes vital to cellular protection and immune regulation.[10]

MECHANISMS OF GLN-MEDIATED PROTECTION
GLN and Cellular/Organ Protection

It is well established that a central component of GLN's beneficial effects involves induction of HSPs, specifically HSP-70.[14–16] Expression of HSPs provides stress tolerance and protection from continued injury that could otherwise cause cell death or impaired recovery.[17] Data show that the stress tolerance provided by HSP-70 can protect against cellular injury, lung injury, ischemia-reperfusion injury, and septic shock.[18] Expression of HSP-70 is dependent on adequate GLN concentrations. GLN-deficient organisms, such as critically ill patients, seem not capable of generating an adequate HSP response.[19,20]

Experiments performed in the authors' laboratory have shown that the mechanism for GLN-mediated induction of HSP-70 is via the hexosamine biosynthetic pathway or O-GlcNAc pathway.[21,22] The O-GlcNAc pathway is know to modify key stress-response proteins to prevent their ubiquitinization and activate transcription factors required for cell survival after injury.[23] GLN is the rate-limiting substrate for the O-GlcNAc pathway.[23] GLN seems to use the O-GlcNAc pathway to induce HSP gene expression via modification and nuclear translocation of key HSP pathway transcription factors, Sp1 and heat shock factor-1 (HSF-1).[21,22] Due to the ability of O-GlcNAc to respond quickly to stress by modifying proteins, it seems part of an early GLN-mediated cellular protective response.

Data from the authors' laboratory show that GLN can induce HSP expression in in vitro, in vivo, and clinical critical care settings. GLN induces HSP-70 expression in intestinal epithelial cells leading to protection against oxidant and heat injury.[24] Using HSF-1 knockout cells[15] and HSP-70 knockout animals, the authors' laboratory showed that the capacity to express HSPs is required for GLN to be protective against cellular injury and that administering GLN to critically ill patients enhances HSP expression and improves clinically relevant outcomes.[25]

GLN and the Inflammatory Response

GLN attenuates the release of proinflammatory cytokines after illness or injury in in vitro and in vivo models.[26,27] Attenuation of the systemic inflammatory response syndrome response seems to correlate with improved survival after infection.[28] Using an experimental model of infection after surgery, acute early administration of GLN and the subsequent HSP induction can attenuate the acute hyperinflammatory response and the massive cytokine release that follows injury or surgery. Specifically, the release of interleukin (IL)-6 and tumor necrosis factor (TNF)-α is attenuated at 6 hours post surgery or injury. The mechanism of this reduced hyperinflammatory response is GLN-mediated attenuation of nuclear binding/activation of nuclear factor κB (NF-κB).[29] The authors' laboratory found that in models of experimental sepsis, 0.75 g/kg of GLN can attenuate nuclear binding/activation of NF-κB and prevent degradation of IκBα, its inhibitory protein.[29]

Data show that GLN's anti-inflammatory effect may be related to HSP expression. In the authors' laboratory, HSP-70 knockout mice (mice having a deletion of the HSP-70 gene) do not demonstrate the aforementioned attenuation of NF-κB after GLN treatment nor do they exhibit attenuation of TNF-α or IL-6.

GLN and Cellular Metabolism/Apoptosis

In work related to cellular metabolism and mitochondrial function, the authors' laboratory has shown that GLN preserves tissue level metabolic function (adenosine triphosphate [ATP]/adenosine diphosphate levels and nicotinamide adenine dinucleotide levels) in the face of sepsis, shock, and ischemia-reperfusion injury.[18] This seems linked to enhanced HSP expression.[18] GLN resuscitation in hemorrhagic shock may restore hepatic ATP levels, according to a recently published study.[30]

According to recent in vitro studies, GLN plays a role in prevention of apoptosis after stress or injury.[31,32] One way GLN may help prevent apoptosis is through the extracellular signal-regulated kinase signaling pathway.[33] This same group also discovered that the phosphoinositide-3 kinase/Akt pathway is activated during starvation. This likely protects cells from apoptosis in times of stress. This further supports the hypothesis that intracellular GLN levels may function as a communicator of stress.

GLN and Immune Function

GLN also influences immune cell regulation. Lymphocytes and macrophages metabolize GLN at a high rate. GLN is needed for the synthesis of purines and pyrimidines, building blocks that become instantly essential when lymphocytes or macrophages are activated. Expression of cell surface activation markers, CD25 (IL-2 receptor α chain), CD45RO (leukocyte common antigen), and CD71 (transferring receptor), are dependent on the presence of GLN.[34] GLN is also required for TNF-α production.[34] Monocyte function is also hindered in the GLN-deficient environment. Altered monocyte major histocompatibility complex class II is associated with postoperative infection and sepsis and linked to expression levels of human leukocyte antigen on DR locus (HLA-DR expression) in cell studies.[34]

Insulin Resistance and Hyperglycemia

Hyperglycemia and insulin resistance contribute to mortality in critical care. At least one clinical trial of GLN in the ICU setting has observed that GLN supplementation improved parameters of hyperglycemia and led to a significant reduction in the number of patients requiring insulin.[35] A separate study set out to study insulin resistance in trauma patients.[36] Forty patients were randomized to receive GLN (0.4 g/kg) or an isocaloric/nitrogenous control supplement. Insulin sensitivity was measured via insulin clamp on days 4 and 8. It was found that the GLN-supplemented patients had the most improved insulin sensitivity.[36] In light of these data, it is reasonable to conclude that some of GLN's beneficial effects may be through insulin-dependent glucose metabolism.

GLN AND CLINICAL OUTCOME IN CRITICAL ILLNESS

In 2002, Novak and colleagues[37] reviewed all trials of GLN therapy in critical illness published until that time. Recent trials of GLN in critical illness have been added to this work, and the updated meta-analysis is available at http://www.criticalcarenutrition.com. According to the results of the new meta-analysis (updated January 31, 2009), enteral or intravenous GLN significantly reduced mortality (RR 0.75; 95% CI, 0.61–0.93; $P = .008$) (**Table 1**) and infectious morbidity (RR 0.79; 95% CI, 0.68–0.93; $P = .005$) (**Table 2**). GLN administration also led to an impressive 2.6-day (95% CI, -4.39 to -0.74; $P = .006$) decrease in ICU length of stay (**Table 3**). In-depth analysis of the many (36) trials included in this analysis reveals that larger doses of GLN (>0.3 g/kg per day) are most effective, and patients receiving parenteral (vs enteral) GLN receive the most benefits. In the subgroup of patients requiring parenteral nutrition, GLN led to a 29% reduction in the risk of death (RR 0.71; CI, 0.55–0.92; $P = .008$) (**Table 4**).

GLN AND PATIENTS WITH HEAD INJURIES

Until recently, there were few data related to GLN feeding and head injury. A study from a research group in China studied the effect of parenteral alanyl-GLN dipeptide (a more stable, soluble form of GLN available worldwide) on the clinical outcomes of patients who sustained severe traumatic brain injury. This large, randomized trial of 46 patients showed a reduction in gastrointestinal hemorrhage, lung infection, and mortality in the group supplemented with GLN.[38]

Berg and colleagues[39,40] published 2 trials dispelling any concerns over GLN crossing the blood-brain barrier and leading to increases in intracerebral levels of glutamate, an excitatory neurotransmitter. In these trials, administering clinically relevant doses of GLN to patients with head injuries did not alter intracerebral glutamate concentrations. Plasma GLN levels were increased after GLN infusion; however, no changes were observed in microdialysate fluid glutamate concentration in the group or in any individual patients.[39]

SUMMARY

GLN has been shown to be a key pharmaconutrient in the body's response to stress and injury. It exerts its protective effects via multiple mechanisms, including direct

Table 1
Effect of enteral and parenteral glutamine on overall mortality in critical illness

Study or Sub-category	Glutamine (n/N)	Control (n/N)	RR (Random) (95% CI)	Weight (%)	RR (Random) (95% CI)	Year
Griffiths	18/42	25/42		23.68	0.72 (0.47, 1.11)	1997
Houdijk	4/41	3/39		2.13	1.27 (0.30, 5.31)	1998
Jones	10/26	9/24		8.66	1.03 (0.50, 2.08)	1999
Powell-Tuck	14/83	20/85		11.63	0.72 (0.39, 1.32)	1999
Brantley	0/31	0/41			Not estimable	2000
Wischmeyer	2/15	5/16		1.99	0.43 (0.10, 1.88)	2001
Garrel	2/21	12/24		2.30	0.19 (0.05, 0.76)	2003
Hall	27/179	30/184		19.12	0.93 (0.57, 1.49)	2003
Zhou	0/20	0/20			Not estimable	2003
Fuentes-Orozco	2/17	3/16		1.59	0.63 (0.12, 3.28)	2004
Xian-Li	0/20	3/21		0.52	0.15 (0.01, 2.73)	2004
Dechelotte 2006	2/58	2/56		1.18	0.97 (0.14, 6.62)	2006
Palmese	6/42	8/42		4.65	0.75 (0.28, 1.97)	2006
Sahin	2/20	6/20		2.00	0.33 (0.08, 1.46)	2007
Cai	17/55	20/55		15.66	0.85 (0.50, 1.44)	2008
Duska	2/10	0/10		0.51	5.00 (0.27, 92.62)	2008
Estivariz	1/32	6/31		1.03	0.16 (0.02, 1.27)	2008
Fuentes-Orozco 2008	2/22	5/22		1.86	0.40 (0.09, 1.85)	2008
Luo 2008	1/23	0/9		0.45	1.25 (0.06, 28.15)	2008
McQuiggan	0/10	2/10		0.51	0.20 (0.01, 3.70)	2008
Perez-Barcena	3/15	0/15		0.53	7.00 (0.39, 124.83)	2008
Total (95% CI)	782	782		100.00	0.75 (0.61, 0.93)	

Total events: 115 (glutamine), 159 (control)
Test for heterogeneity: χ^2 = 16.81, df = 18 (P = .54), I^2 = 0%
Test for overall effect: z = 2.65 (P = .008)

0.1 0.2 0.5 1 2 5 10
Favours glutamine   Favours control

Table 2
Effect of enteral and parenteral glutamine on infectious complications

Study or Sub-category	Glutamine (n/N)	Control (n/N)	RR (Random) (95% CI)	Weight (%)	RR (Random) (95% CI)	Year
Griffiths	28/42	26/42		17.16	1.08 (0.78, 1.48)	1997
Houdijk	20/35	26/37		14.79	0.81 (0.57, 1.16)	1998
Wischmeyer	7/12	9/14		6.02	0.91 (0.49, 1.68)	2001
Hall	38/179	43/184		13.15	0.91 (0.62, 1.33)	2003
Zhou	2/20	6/20		1.16	0.33 (0.08, 1.46)	2003
Fuentes-Orozco	4/17	12/16		3.00	0.31 (0.13, 0.77)	2004
Zhou 2004	3/15	4/15		1.46	0.75 (0.20, 2.79)	2004
Dechelotte 2006	23/58	32/56		12.87	0.69 (0.47, 1.03)	2006
Palmese	2/42	6/42		1.07	0.33 (0.07, 1.56)	2006
Estivariz	13/30	16/29		7.99	0.79 (0.46, 1.33)	2008
Fuentes-Orozco 2008	9/22	16/22		7.06	0.56 (0.32, 0.99)	2008
Perez-Barcena	11/15	13/15		14.28	0.85 (0.59, 1.22)	2008
Total (95% CI)	487	492		100.00	0.79 (0.68, 0.93)	

Total events: 160 (glutamine), 209 (control)
Test for heterogeneity: $\chi^2 = 13.14$, df = 11 ($P = .28$), $I^2 = 16.3\%$
Test for overall effect: $z = 2.81$ ($P = .005$)

0.1   0.2   0.5   1   2   5   10

Favours glutamine   Favours control

Table 3

Effect of enteral and parenteral glutamine administration on length of stay

Study or Sub-category	N	Glutamine (Mean [SD])	N	Control (Mean [SD])	WMD (Random) (95% CI)	WMD (Random) (95% CI)	Weight (%)	Year
Houdijk	35	32.70(17.10)	37	33.00(23.80)		−0.30 (−9.83, 9.23)	2.83	1998
Powell-Tuck	83	43.40(34.10)	85	48.90(38.40)		−5.50 (−16.48, 5.48)	2.26	1999
Brantley	31	19.50(8.80)	41	20.80(11.50)		−1.30 (−5.99, 3.39)	6.87	2000
Wischmeyer	12	40.00(10.00)	14	40.00(9.00)		0.00 (−7.36, 7.36)	4.12	2001
Zhou	20	67.00(4.00)	20	73.00(6.00)		−6.00 (−9.16, −2.84)	9.14	2003
Fuentes-Orozco	17	16.50(8.90)	16	16.70(7.00)		−0.20 (−5.65, 5.25)	5.93	2004
Peng	25	46.59(12.98)	23	55.68(17.36)		−9.09 (−17.82, −0.36)	3.24	2004
Zhou 2004	15	42.00(7.00)	15	46.00(6.60)		−4.00 (−8.87, 0.87)	6.64	2004
Palmese	42	12.00(4.60)	42	13.00(3.40)		−1.00 (−2.73, 0.73)	11.32	2006
Sahin	20	14.20(4.40)	20	16.40(3.90)		−2.20 (−4.78, 0.38)	10.07	2007
Cai	55	22.10(4.90)	55	23.80(5.10)		−1.70 (−3.57, 0.17)	11.13	2008
Estivariz	15	20.00(2.00)	12	30.00(6.00)		−10.00 (−13.54, −6.46)	8.54	2008
Fuentes-Orozco 2008	22	30.18(10.42)	22	26.59(13.30)		3.59 (−3.47, 10.65)	4.36	2008
Luo 2008	11	7.60(0.70)	9	6.90(0.90)		0.70 (−0.02, 1.42)	12.36	2008
McQuiggan	10	32.00(13.60)	10	39.30(36.30)		−7.30 (−31.33, 16.73)	0.55	2008
Perez-Barcena	15	35.50(33.60)	15	42.90(28.80)		−7.40 (−29.80, 15.00)	0.63	2008
Total (95% CI)	428		436			−2.56 (−4.39, −0.74)	100.00	
Test for heterogeneity: χ^2 = 62.15, df = 15 (P<.00001), I^2 = 75.9%								
Test for overall effect: z = 2.76 (P = .006)								

−10   −5   0   5   10

Favours glutamine   Favours control

Table 4
Effect of parenteral glutamine on mortality

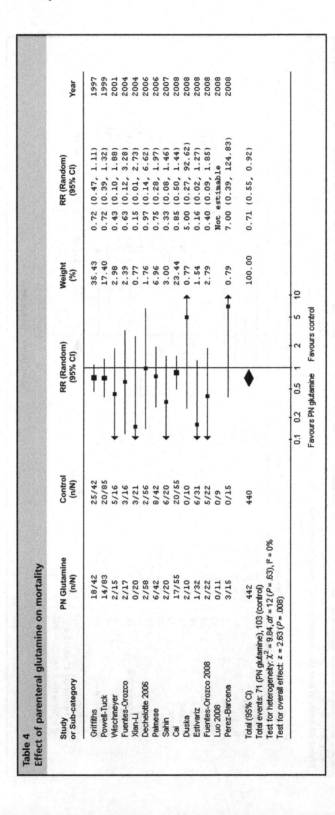

Study or Sub-category	PN Glutamine (n/N)	Control (n/N)	RR (Random) (95% CI)	Weight (%)	RR (Random) (95% CI)	Year
Griffiths	18/42	25/42		35.43	0.72 (0.47, 1.11)	1997
Powell-Tuck	14/83	20/85		17.40	0.72 (0.39, 1.32)	1999
Wischmeyer	2/15	5/16		2.98	0.43 (0.10, 1.88)	2001
Fuentes-Orozco	2/17	3/16		2.39	0.63 (0.12, 3.28)	2004
Xian-Li	0/20	3/21		0.77	0.15 (0.01, 2.73)	2004
Dechelotte 2006	2/58	2/56		1.76	0.97 (0.14, 6.62)	2006
Palmese	6/42	8/42		6.96	0.75 (0.28, 1.97)	2006
Sahin	2/20	6/20		3.00	0.33 (0.08, 1.46)	2007
Cai	17/55	20/55		23.44	0.85 (0.50, 1.44)	2008
Duska	2/10	0/10		0.77	5.00 (0.27, 92.62)	2008
Estivariz	1/32	6/31		1.54	0.16 (0.02, 1.27)	2008
Fuentes-Orozco 2008	2/22	5/22		2.79	0.40 (0.09, 1.85)	2008
Luo 2008	0/11	0/9			Not estimable	2008
Perez-Barcena	3/15	0/15		0.79	7.00 (0.39, 124.83)	2008
Total (95% CI)	442	440		100.00	0.71 (0.55, 0.92)	

Total events: 71 (PN glutamine), 103 (control)
Test for heterogeneity: $X^2 = 9.84$, $df = 12$ ($P = .63$), $I^2 = 0\%$
Test for overall effect: $z = 2.63$ ($P = .008$)

0.1 0.2 0.5 1 2 5 10

Favours PN glutamine   Favours control

protection of cells and tissue from injury, attenuation of inflammation, and preservation of metabolic function. Data support GLN as an ideal pharmacologic intervention to prevent or treat MODS after sepsis or other injuries in the ICU population. These data are supported clinically by a large and growing body of data showing that in well-defined critically ill patient groups GLN can be a life-saving intervention.

The final answer as to whether or not GLN should be used routinely in ICUs will come after the current ongoing clinical trials are completed. The large amount of mechanistic data and translational evidence on the use of GLN in ICUs has led to increased funding of clinical trials of GLN. The Reducing Deaths due to Oxidant Stress trial group has begun clinical trials in Canada, the United States, and Europe after an extensive published pilot trial that was completed in 2007.[41] This study implements a factorial design to examine the effects of GLN and antioxidants on mortality in the ICU setting and collects biologic specimens to help elucidate mechanistic pathways.

Currently, the clinical nutrition guidelines of every major nutrition and critical care society give intravenous GLN a grade A recommendation for use in critically ill patients requiring parenteral nutrition.[42,43] The data from these societies and the current meta-analysis indicate larger-dose (>0.35–0.5 g/kg per day of actual GLN) intravenous administration is where the clear mortality benefit occurs.[37] Based on clinical and laboratory data, studies giving lower doses of GLN are unlikely to provide benefit because doses below 0.35 to 0.5 g/kg do not serve to correct the marked GLN deficiency seen in critical illness. Furthermore, lower doses are not shown to induce the mechanistic benefits hypothesized for GLN's benefits.[16]

Thus, in ICU patients requiring parenteral nutrition, "the time has come, the time is now" for routine use of high-dose (>0.35 g/kg per day) GLN therapy. In other patient groups, large ongoing trials of GLN in critical illness will reveal if the time will come for GLN to be recommended as standard of care for all ICU patients.

REFERENCES

1. Martin GS, Mannino DM, Eaton S, et al. The epidemiology of sepsis in the United States from 1979 through 2000. N Engl J Med 2003;348(16):1546–54.
2. Murphy SL. Deaths: final data for 1998. Natl Vital Stat Rep 2000;48(11):1–105.
3. Dombrovskiy VY, Martin AA, Sunderram J, et al. Rapid increase in hospitalization and mortality rates for severe sepsis in the United States: a trend analysis from 1993 to 2003. Crit Care Med 2007;35(5):1244–50.
4. Rangel-Frausto MS, Pittet D, Costigan M, et al. The natural history of the systemic inflammatory response syndrome (SIRS). A prospective study. JAMA 1995; 273(2):117–23.
5. Fink MP. Cytopathic hypoxia. Is oxygen use impaired in sepsis as a result of an acquired intrinsic derangement in cellular respiration? Crit Care Clin 2002; 18(1):165–75.
6. Gamrin L, Essen P, Forsberg AM, et al. A descriptive study of skeletal muscle metabolism in critically ill patients: free amino acids, energy-rich phosphates, protein, nucleic acids, fat, water, and electrolytes. Crit Care Med 1996;24(4): 575–83.
7. Newsholme EA, Crabtree B, Ardawi MS. Glutamine metabolism in lymphocytes: its biochemical, physiological and clinical importance. Q J Exp Physiol 1985; 70(4):473–89.
8. Wilmore DW. The effect of glutamine supplementation in patients following elective surgery and accidental injury. J Nutr 2001;131(Suppl 9):2543S–9 [discussion: 2550S–1S].

9. Oudemans-van Straaten HM, Bosman RJ, Treskes M, et al. Plasma glutamine depletion and patient outcome in acute ICU admissions. Intensive Care Med 2001;27(1):84–90.

10. Wischmeyer PE. Glutamine: role in critical illness and ongoing clinical trials. Curr Opin Gastroenterol 2008;24(2):190–7.

11. Coeffier M, Dechelotte P. The role of glutamine in intensive care unit patients: mechanisms of action and clinical outcome. Nutr Rev 2005;63(2):65–9.

12. Preiser JC, Wernerman J. Glutamine, a life-saving nutrient, but why? Crit Care Med 2003;31(10):2555–6.

13. Curi R, Newsholme P, Procopio J, et al. Glutamine, gene expression, and cell function. Front Biosci 2007;12:344–57.

14. Wischmeyer PE. Glutamine and heat shock protein expression. Nutrition 2002; 18(3):225–8.

15. Morrison AL, Dinges M, Singleton KD, et al. Glutamine's protection against cellular injury is dependent on heat shock factor-1. Am J Phys Cell Physiol 2006;290(6):C1625–32.

16. Wischmeyer PE. Glutamine: the first clinically relevant pharmacological regulator of heat shock protein expression? Curr Opin Clin Nutr Metab Care 2006;9(3): 201–6.

17. Pelham HR. Speculations on the functions of the major heat shock and glucose-regulated proteins. Cell 1986;46(7):959–61.

18. Weitzel LR, Mayles WJ, Sandoval PA, et al. Effects of pharmaconutrients on cellular dysfunction and the microcirculation in critical illness. Curr Opin Anaesthesiol 2009;22(2):177–83.

19. Weiss YG, Bouwman A, Gehan B, et al. Cecal ligation and double puncture impairs heat shock protein 70 (HSP-70) expression in the lungs of rats. Shock 2000;13(1):19–23.

20. Singleton KD, Serkova N, Beckey VE, et al. Glutamine attenuates lung injury and improves survival after sepsis: role of enhanced heat shock protein expression. Crit Care Med 2005;33(6):1206–13.

21. Singleton KD, Wischmeyer PE. Glutamine induces heat shock protein expression via O-glycosylation and phosphorylation of HSF-1 and Sp1. JPEN J Parenter Enteral Nutr 2008;32(4):371–6.

22. Hamiel CR, Pinto S, Hau A, et al. Glutamine enhances heat shock protein 70 expression via increased hexosamine biosynthetic pathway activity. Am J Physiol Cell Physiol 2009;297(6):C1509–19.

23. Zachara NE, Hart GW. Cell signaling, the essential role of O-GlcNAc! Biochim Biophys Acta 2006;1761(5–6):599–617.

24. Wischmeyer PE, Musch MW, Madonna MB, et al. Glutamine protects intestinal epithelial cells: role of inducible HSP70. Am J Physiol 1997;272(4 Pt 1):G879–84.

25. Ziegler TR, Ogden LG, Singleton KD, et al. Parenteral glutamine increases serum heat shock protein 70 in critically ill patients. Intensive Care Med 2005;31(8): 1079–86.

26. Lappas GD, Karl IE, Hotchkiss RS. Effect of ethanol and sodium arsenite on HSP-72 formation and on survival in a murine endotoxin model. Shock 1994;2(1):34–9 [discussion: 40].

27. Villar J, Edelson JD, Post M, et al. Induction of heat stress proteins is associated with decreased mortality in an animal model of acute lung injury. Am Rev Respir Dis 1993;147(1):177–81.

28. Chu EK, Ribeiro SP, Slutsky AS. Heat stress increases survival rates in lipopolysaccharide-stimulated rats. Crit Care Med 1997;25(10):1727–32.

29. Singleton KD, Beckey VE, Wischmeyer PE. Glutamine prevents activation of nf-kappab and stress kinase pathways, attenuates inflammatory cytokine release, and prevents acute respiratory distress syndrome (ARDS) following sepsis. Shock 2005;24(6):583–9.

30. Fan J, Li Y, Levy RM, et al. Hemorrhagic shock induces NAD(P)H oxidase activation in neutrophils: role of HMGB1–TLR4 signaling. J Immunol 2007;178(10): 6573–80.

31. Evans ME, Jones DP, Ziegler TR. Glutamine inhibits cytokine-induced apoptosis in human colonic epithelial cells via the pyrimidine pathway. Am J Physiol Gastrointest Liver Physiol 2005;289(3):G388–96.

32. Paquette JC, Guerin PJ, Gauthier ER. Rapid induction of the intrinsic apoptotic pathway by L-glutamine starvation. J Cell Physiol 2005;202(3):912–21.

33. Larson SD, Li J, Chung DH, et al. Molecular mechanisms contributing to glutamine-mediated intestinal cell survival. Am J Physiol Gastrointest Liver Physiol 2007;293(6):G1262–71.

34. Roth E. Nonnutritive effects of glutamine. J Nutr 2008;138(10):2025S–31.

35. Dechelotte P, Hasselmann M, Cynober L, et al. L-alanyl-L-glutamine dipeptide-supplemented total parenteral nutrition reduces infectious complications and glucose intolerance in critically ill patients: the French controlled, randomized, double-blind, multicenter study. Crit Care Med 2006;34(3):598–604.

36. Bakalar B, Duska F, Pachl J, et al. Parenterally administered dipeptide alanyl-glutamine prevents worsening of insulin sensitivity in multiple-trauma patients. Crit Care Med 2006;34(2):381–6.

37. Novak F, Heyland DK, Avenell A, et al. Glutamine supplementation in serious illness: a systematic review of the evidence. Crit Care Med 2002;30(9):2022–9.

38. Yang DL, Xu JF. Effect of dipeptide of glutamine and alanine on severe traumatic brain injury. Clin J Traumatool 2007;10:145–9.

39. Berg A, Bellander BM, Wanecek M, et al. Intravenous glutamine supplementation to head trauma patients leaves cerebral glutamate concentration unaffected. Intensive Care Med 2006;32(11):1741–6.

40. Berg A, Bellander BM, Wanecek M, et al. The pattern of amino acid exchange across the brain is unaffected by intravenous glutamine supplementation in head trauma patients. Clin Nutr 2008;27(6):816–21.

41. Heyland DKDR, Day A, et al. Optimizing the dose of glutamine dipeptides and anitoxidants in critically ill patients: a phase I dose-finding study. JPEN J Parenter Enteral Nutr 2007;31:109–18.

42. McClave SA, Martindale RG, Vanek VW, et al. Guidelines for the provision and assessment of nutrition support therapy in the adult critically ill patient: Society of Critical Care Medicine (SCCM) and American Society for Parenteral and Enteral Nutrition (A.S.P.E.N. JPEN J Parenter Enteral Nutr 2009;33(3):277–316.

43. Singer P, Berger MM, Van den Berghe G, et al. ESPEN guidelines on parenteral nutrition: intensive care. Clin Nutr 2009;28(4):387–400.

Enhanced Recovery After Surgery: The Future of Improving Surgical Care

Krishna K. Varadhan, MSc, MRCS[a], Dileep N. Lobo, DM, FRCS[a],
Olle Ljungqvist, MD, PhD[b],*

KEYWORDS

- Enhanced recovery • Surgery • Fast track • Colorectal surgery
- Outcome • Hospital stay • Complications • Traditional care

Enhanced recovery after surgery (ERAS) is a multimodal perioperative care pathway designed to attenuate the stress response during the patients' journey through a surgical procedure (**Fig. 1**) to facilitate the maintenance of preoperative bodily compositions and organ function and in doing so achieve early recovery. The concept of multimodal surgical care was pioneered in the late 1990s by Professor Henrik Kehlet in Copenhagen. He envisaged the need for improvement in various elements of hospital health care systems, targeted at specific medical concerns of various subsets of patients and all patients undergoing surgery, so that the overall outcome could be improved.[1] This process was initially thought to be a radical move away from tradition and dogma to a fundamental change in the perioperative management of patients and struggled to gain wider acceptance. However, with accumulating evidence from several randomized controlled trials (RCTs), systematic reviews,[2] and meta-analyses of the effects of the individual elements of ERAS pathway,[3–5] significant benefits of the individual elements were identified and an evidence-based consensus protocol for perioperative care in patients undergoing colonic surgery was drafted by

Conflict of interest: D.N.L. and O.L. are members of the ERAS Group and have received research funding/honoraria/travel bursaries from Nutricia Clinical Care and Fresenius Kabi. O.L. is also the holder of a patent for a preoperative carbohydrate drink, licensed to Nutricia for manufacture. K.K.V. has no conflict of interest to declare.

Funding: K.K.V. was supported by a research fellowship awarded by the Nottingham Digestive Diseases Centre NIHR Biomedical Research Unit.

[a] Division of Gastrointestinal Surgery, Nottingham Digestive Diseases Centre NIHR Biomedical Research Unit, Nottingham University Hospitals, Queen's Medical Centre, Nottingham NG7 2UH, UK

[b] Department of Surgery, Örebro University Hospital, SE-701 85 Örebro, Sweden

* Corresponding author.

E-mail address: olle.ljungqvist@ki.se

Crit Care Clin 26 (2010) 527–547

doi:10.1016/j.ccc.2010.04.003

0749-0704/10/$ – see front matter © 2010 Elsevier Inc. All rights reserved.

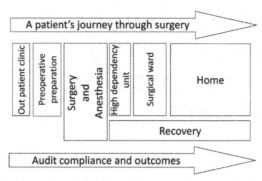

Fig. 1. A patient's journey through an operative procedure.

the ERAS Group in 2005.[6] This document ushered in a paradigm shift in perioperative care and the evidence base was updated in 2009[7] to include rectal surgery. The key factors that keep patients in the hospital after uncomplicated major abdominal surgery include the need for parenteral analgesia, intravenous fluids secondary to persistent gut dysfunction, and bed rest caused by lack of mobility. These factors often overlap and interact to delay recovery and discharge from the hospital. The key elements of the ERAS pathways are aimed to address these issues and the interventions that facilitate early recovery cover all three phases of the perioperative period during the patients' journey. They also provide clear guidance to all members of the clinical team, namely anesthetists, surgeons, physiotherapists, dietitians, and nursing staff.

HISTORY AND PHILOSOPHY OF ENHANCED RECOVERY AFTER SURGERY

The main philosophy of the ERAS protocol is to reduce the metabolic stress caused by surgical trauma and at the same time support the return of functions that allow patients to get back to normal activities rapidly (**Fig. 2**).

The work by Henrik Kehlet in 1997[1] proposed a multimodal approach to perioperative care to achieve this goal. A couple of years later, the same group published a paper reporting median length of stay of 2 days following colonic resections using this philosophy.[8] These were followed by similar reports from the United States.[9]

In 2001 Fearon and Ljungqvist assembled leading surgical groups to form the Enhanced Recovery After Surgery Study Group. The idea was to further develop the protocol initiated by Kehlet and coworkers and to also have several international surgical units use the same perioperative protocol. This idea would then enable a solid basis for clinical trials to further improve the concept and to allow studies of yet unanswered questions to be addressed in a multinational, multicenter setting.

The Groups spent about 1 year to scrutinize the literature and to update the previous protocols used by Kehlet's group. This protocol was later published.[6] When assembling the perioperative protocols in use in the various units, it became clear that different practices were being used and that each unit was using about 30% to 40% of what had been found to be best practice in the literature.[10] This finding inspired the group to perform a survey of practices in use in the countries involved and again different and mostly outdated treatments of the traditional kind were in use throughout Northern Europe.[11,12] Given the vast gap between the best practice according to the evidence available and what was in use, and the fact that the different units often had different traditions, it was decided to study the period of change into

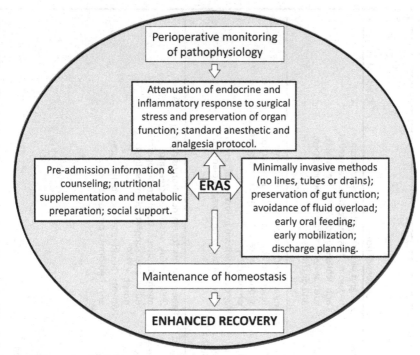

Fig. 2. Philosophy of ERAS.

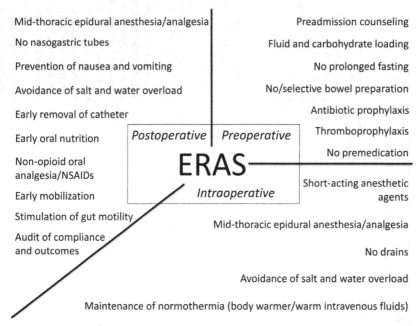

Fig. 3. Components of ERAS.

Table 1
Summary of preoperative recommendations

Preoperative Elements	Rationale	Recommendations	Grade of Evidence
Preadmission information and counseling	Preadmission counseling ensures a clear understanding of the intended perioperative care to be received with emphasis on attaining specific preset targets and would help in alleviating the stress responses to surgery.[21–23,27,28]	Oral and written patient information regarding hospitalization, pain relief, and achieving postoperative targets, such as early nutrition, mobilization, and discharge	C
No bowel preparation	Bowel preparation leads to dehydration and changes in fluid and electrolyte balance.[17] No change[25] or rather an increased risk for complications, such as prolonged postoperative, and increased risk for anastomotic leakage from mechanical bowel preparation.[26,30,31,33]	Patients undergoing elective colonic resection above peritoneal reflection should not receive routine oral bowel preparation. May be considered in low rectal resection where a diverting stoma is planned.[77]	A
Preoperative nutritional support	Approximately 27%–45% of hospitalized patients are malnourished.[29,32,81] Increases risk for tissue wasting, impaired immune function, impaired healing, and organ dysfunction resulting in increased morbidity, length of stay, readmission rates, delayed recovery, hospital costs, and mortality.[20,24,73] Preoperative carbohydrate loading reduces the incidence of complications[34,48] and facilitates accelerated recovery through early return of gut function and shorter hospital stay leading to an improved perioperative well being.[51,52,54]	Patients at risk for malnutrition using NRS 2002 or SGA, or similar screening methods, should be given preoperative nutritional support, given orally if possible.[83,85] Patients should receive carbohydrate-enriched drinks preoperatively.[7]	A

Preoperative fasting	Preoperative fasting and surgery predisposes to metabolic stress and insulin resistance.[72] Overnight fasting does not reduce the risk for aspiration. Intake of clear fluids until 2 hours before anesthesia is as safe.[74]	The consensus guidelines from a Cochrane review[74] and guidelines from anesthetic societies recommend clear fluids until 2 hours before induction of anesthesia and a 6-hour fast for solid food.[7]	A
No long-acting sedatives/premedication	Long-acting sedatives, hypnotics, and opioids (preemptive analgesia) were thought to reduce anxiety and stress related to surgery, but these effects are far outweighed by the risk for prolonged recovery caused by inability to drink or mobilize postoperatively. No effect on postoperative pain relief by starting analgesic treatment before the operation.[50] Short-acting anxiolytics have not shown prolonged recovery or length of stay.[53]	Medications causing long-term sedation should be avoided. Short-acting medications given to facilitate insertion of epidural catheter are acceptable.	A
Antimicrobial Prophylaxis	Prophylactic antibiotics minimize infectious complications in colorectal surgery.[78]	A single dose, 1 hour before skin incision and further doses for procedures lasting more than 3 hours.[78]	A
Thromboembolic prophylaxis	Increased risk for thromboembolic complications in certain high-risk patients undergoing major abdominal surgery is associated with prolonged hospitalization and recovery.	Subcutaneous low-dose unfractionated heparin or subcutaneous low-molecular-weight heparin.[76,80]	C

Abbreviations: NRS, nutritional risk screening; SGA, subjective global assessment.

Table 2
Summary of intraoperative recommendations

Intraoperative Elements	Rationale	Recommendations	Grade of Evidence
Standard anesthetic protocol/mid-thoracic epidural with local anesthetic/opioid	Rational use of short-acting agents to facilitate proactive recovery postoperatively. Preoperative commencement of mid-thoracic epidural blocks stress hormone release and attenuates postoperative insulin resistance.[7] Helps in achieving analgesia and sympathetic blockade and in preventing gut paralysis.[49]	Avoid long-acting opioids. Mid-thoracic epidural commenced preoperatively, containing local anesthetic in combination with a low-dose opioid. Consider short-acting inhalational anesthesia as an alternative to total intravenous anesthesia.	A
Laparoscopic/minimally invasive surgery	Decreased inflammatory response, insulin resistance, improved pulmonary function, early return of bowel function, mobilization, less pain, reduced incidence of complications, readmissions, and length of stay.[38,45,46]	Laparoscopic-assisted colorectal surgery is recommended in dedicated specialist centers, with outcomes comparable to open surgery.	A
Maintenance of normothermia	Reduced wound infections, cardiac complications, bleeding, and transfusion requirements.[35,37,41,43,44]	Routine use of upper-body, forced-air heating cover; prevention of hypothermia by warm intravenous fluids	A
Perioperative fluid management	Sodium and fluid overload delays return of gastrointestinal function, prolongs hospital stay, increases side-effects and complications.[39,40,42]	Fluid restriction, avoiding hypovolemia, sodium, and fluid overload Goal-directed fluid therapy in high-risk cases	A
Selective use of drains	Routine use of drains does not reduce the incidence or severity of anastomotic leak.[36,69]	No drains after routine colonic resections above peritoneal reflections Short-term (<24 hours) drainage after low anterior resections	A
Urinary drainage	Increased risk for urinary tract infections following prolonged use.[70] Reduced incidence of complications[58]	Suprapubic catheter for rectal surgery Early removal of catheters following colonic surgery	C

modern and evidence-based care in more detail. A database was initiated where the demographics of the patients were to be recorded and detailed information about the surgery and the perioperative care were also noted. A vast amount of work was put into defining complications and having them recorded. The same was true for many other details, in particular the definitions of a given surgical procedure that could be different in different units. The physiological and operative severity score for the enumeration of mortality and morbidity (POSSUM) scoring system was also included along with the American Society of Anesthesiologists (ASA) classification to give an opportunity to compare different units with different patient populations. One of the criticisms of Kehlet's first report was that there had been patient selection. When comparing the units using the POSSUM scoring, the patient material was remarkably similar in Copenhagen, Tromsö, Stockholm, Maastricht, and Edinburgh.

Each unit went ahead and started the implementation of the new routines. The ERAS study group met on a regular basis and reviewed the data and shared experiences. It became obvious that all units had difficulties getting the new program in place, but the problems were not always the same. Although one unit may have problems overcoming resistance for a change in practice, the fact that another unit was using that treatment successfully often helped effect the change. Already during the first periods of running the program it became evident that the Copenhagen group was much ahead of the rest and that it would take some time to catch up with them. They, therefore, left the collaboration after the initial phase. It was also clear that the patient material was much the same in all units and thus it should be possible to have patients recover in about 3 days to be ready for discharge in all units. The Copenhagen group, having sent patients home on day 2 as the target, had a high readmission rate of 25%, whereas the rest had a readmission rate of around 10% after a hospital stay of 3 to 4 days. This result led to the Copenhagen group to change the targeted stay to 3 days. It was, however, obvious that the most important factor for the success of the protocol was the time itself that the program had been in place.[13]

A typical example for the Group was the work done at Ersta hospital in Stockholm. A prospective collection of data was done before the commencement of the program and the data from these patients were later compared with the first 100 patients entering the program. From these data, it was obvious that even if it takes time to put the entire program in place, it is still possible to achieve significant improvements in outcomes and recovery from the start.[14] However, without the use of the database it would have been difficult to detect where the initial problems were and in which units the program did or did not work. But already at the first complete follow-up it became clear that there were two main problems: patients were given too much fluids during and after surgery and the protocol was not working well from time to time at the post-operative high-dependency unit. These issues were addressed and another round of training was performed. Again it was shown that with improved compliance with the protocol, further improvements in outcomes could be achieved. This time complication rates reduced as did several of the key problems that delayed discharge.[15]

The database rapidly grew to one of the largest of its kind and opened possibilities to study the roles of various factors for outcomes. For instance, one report showed that when running an ERAS protocol in daily practice, factors, such as a low body mass index, no longer affected outcomes.[16] Clearly, even vulnerable patients who are at risk also benefit from this standardized protocol and a recent study has shown that patients classified as ASA 3 and 4 can also recover rapidly when managed according to the ERAS protocol.[16] A mixture of patients undergoing colorectal procedures was fit for discharge at a median of 4 days. More

Table 3
Summary of postoperative recommendations

Postoperative Elements	Rationale	Recommendations	Grade of Evidence
No routine use of nasogastric tube	Facilitates earlier return of bowel function. Not associated with increased risk for complications or length of stay.[66,71]	Nasogastric tubes should not be used routinely in the postoperative period. Used in selected cases of postoperative ileus, or unless severe PONV	A
Aggressive treatment of PONV	Facilitates early oral feeding. Symptoms related to postoperative ileus and opioids can be more stressful than postoperative pain. Female gender, nonsmoking status, history of motion sickness or PONV, and postoperative opioids confer high risk.	Individuals at moderate risk (>2 factors) should receive, prophylactically, dexamethasone sodium phosphate at induction or serotonin receptor antagonist at the end of surgery.[75,79]	A
Prevention of postoperative ileus	Surgical stress, opioids, bowel handling, and fluid overload predispose to ileus and impair GI function leading to delayed discharge. Oral magnesium oxide promotes postoperative bowel function.[56,57]	Mid-thoracic epidural analgesia, avoidance of fluid overload, and laparoscopic approach, where possible, is recommended. A low-dose postoperative laxative, such as magnesium oxide, may also be considered.	A
Postoperative analgesia/Mid-thoracic epidural analgesia	TEDA results in better pain relief and earlier return-of-bowel function compared with patient-controlled analgesia.[60,65,67,68] Ineffective pain control, analgesia with oral or intravenous opiates, lack of mobility, and loss of appetite contributes to the delayed GI recovery.[59] TEDA also results in attenuated stress response, insulin resistance, reduced incidence of respiratory and cardiovascular complications.[61]	Continuous epidural mid-thoracic low-dose local anesthetic and opioid combinations for approximately 48 hours, following elective colonic surgery and approximately 72–96 hours after pelvic surgery. Acetaminophen (paracetamol) for baseline analgesia (4g/d) postoperatively. Boluses for breakthrough pain NSAIDS started following removal of epidural (multimodal analgesia). Urinary catheter does not have to stay for full duration of epidural and should be removed at earliest	A

Early oral nutrition	Less gut permeability, early return of bowel function, reduced length of stay and complications.[59,62–64]	Oral diet, day of surgery with nutritional supplements (200 mL, energy dense, 2–3 times daily) until normal food intake is achieved. Continued for several weeks in nutritionally depleted patients.	A
Early mobilization	Decreases insulin resistance, risk of thromboembolism and pulmonary dysfunction. Increases muscle strength and facilitates early discharge.	Encourage independence and mobilization for at least 2 hours on the day of surgery (eg, turning, sitting in bed) and 6 hours thereafter (eg, walking).	C
Discharge criteria	Addressing patients' special needs and anticipating problems delaying discharge facilitates early recovery and does not increase readmission rates.[55]	Criteria for discharge: mobilized to preoperative level, pain control on oral analgesic, return of gut function, and no complications in need of hospital care.	C
Systematic audit	Documenting defined outcomes after implementation of ERAS programs ensures standard of care and identifies areas for improvement.	A systematic audit should be performed to allow direct comparison across institutions.	C

Abbreviations: GI, gastrointestinal; NSAIDs, nonsteroidal antiinflammatory drugs; PONV, postoperative nausea and vomiting; TEDA, thoracic epidural analgesia.

work is needed in this particular field, but given that the protocol itself relies completely on best practice it would seem odd if the most vulnerable patients should have any benefit from not being treated in an optimal way. Another novel advantage of the database is that it has helped provide information about compliance with the various elements of the ERAS pathway and relate this to outcome.[14] Reporting how well various elements of a perioperative protocol have been employed has major impact on outcomes, but this information is something that is almost always missing.

The ERAS study group has recently been expanded with the inclusion of members from Nottingham and St Mark's Hospital in the United Kingdom and from Charité Hospitals in Berlin. The Group has also decided to further expand the network within and outside of Europe. The interest internationally is growing fast and more clinicians are realizing that there are clear advantages to using experiences from other units and from training sessions when trying to implement and spread the use of optimal perioperative care. This mission is one that the Group has now decided to undertake and the ERAS group is now organizing itself to run major training sessions in multiple countries. At the same time the plan is to introduce the database to as many units as possible and to set standards for audit and clinical research. The spreading of best practice will also serve to help form clinical research networks that can further improve the care of this large group of patients.

Most hospitals are organized in smaller units within larger departments and the communication between the different departments is often far from optimal. In particular, it is unusual that staff from one unit are aware of what is actually going on in the unit to which most of their patients are referred. Integration of all the treatments using a multimodal approach at various stages of the patients' journey leads to better outcome.

Fluid administration represents a good example of how things can go wrong in many places leading to problems further down the chain. The surgeon may still be a believer in bowel cleansing and preoperative fasting (although both are shown to be outdated as a routine). Bowel cleansing dehydrates patients[17] and so does overnight fasting, to some extent. Once anesthesia is induced, regardless of whether it is regional or general, the blood pressure will drop. If patients are dehydrated, the pressure will fall even more. This leads to the anesthetist or the nurse giving intravenous fluids to restore the effective circulatory volume. Often patients receive around 3 to 4 L of fluid in excess during a colonic resection lasting 2 to 3 hours. The excess fluid is often followed postoperatively by even more intravenous fluids. Most of this fluid will end up in interstitial space overload in most tissues and organ systems, including the gastrointestinal tract.[18] This practice is one of the main reasons for postoperative ileus that leave patients with abdominal distension, raised intra-abdominal pressure, stretching of the wound, stress on the anastomosis, pain that is often difficult to relieve without large doses of morphine, additional nausea and vomiting, further ileus as a result of that medication, and the vicious cycle is perpetuated.[18,19] It all began with the surgeon ordering the wrong treatments, causing problems for the anesthetist who in turn also orders the wrong treatment. This practice could easily set patients back to stay in the hospital up to 1 week longer, often without the capacity to eat, and hence, losing muscle and strength, which results in a substantially longer convalescence to return to normal function.

The ERAS protocol would have had patients go through the same operation with a completely different protocol and outcome: no bowel cleansing, dinner and drinks on the evening before the operation, carbohydrate drinks 2 hours before anesthesia, and epidural activated in patients who are normovolemic. If there is any fall of blood pressure, the procedure is to limit fluids using colloids and balanced salt solutions according to protocol (typically 1500 mL total) or under guidance of an esophageal Doppler, and if needed, use vasopressors to control blood pressure during surgery. Immediately after surgery patients are encouraged to drink and eat again. The target for the fluid regimen is to have the patients' weight stable through day 1 and to take down the drip the morning after surgery. Several other factors also come into play to secure gut mobility as fast as possible after surgery, but those previously mentioned give the general idea behind the concept.

COMPONENTS OF ENHANCED RECOVERY AFTER SURGERY

Fig. 3 depicts the various elements of the ERAS pathway, which are grouped according to the timing of intervention of these elements throughout the perioperative period. Although most of these elements are derived from high-quality evidence from published literature, some of the less studied elements of the ERAS pathway are based on common consensus review or derived from traditional-care settings.

The rationale[7,17,20–73] for incorporating these elements in the ERAS pathway and the summary of recommendations for individual elements[74–83] with the grades of evidence according to the Center for Evidence Based Medicine, Oxford, England,[84] are illustrated in **Tables 1–3**. **Table 1** shows ERAS elements that are instituted in the preoperative period, whereas **Tables 2** and **3** illustrate the elements that form the ERAS pathway in the intra- and postoperative periods, respectively.

ROLE OF LAPAROSCOPY

Laparoscopic colorectal surgery has struggled to get wider acceptance in ERAS protocols because of its steep learning curve, concerns with oncological outcomes, and initial reports on port-site recurrence after curative resection. Several studies show that these reasons are unjustified and have reported individual advantages of minimally invasive surgery, such as reduced inflammatory response, insulin resistance, improved pulmonary function, early return of bowel function, mobilization, less pain, reduced incidence of complications, and readmissions, leading to shorter hospital stays and early recovery, despite varied postoperative management.[38,45,46] This finding is supported by two meta-analyses and a Cochrane review comparing outcomes of laparoscopic colorectal resections that have reported early return of bowel function; less analgesic requirements; and more importantly, similar oncological clearance, no significant difference in local recurrence, distant metastasis, or port or wound-site recurrence.[86–88] Laparoscopic surgery is associated with earlier return to full activity (approximately 2 weeks, compared with 8 weeks for open surgery) within the ERAS program.[89,90] A study looking at health-related quality-of-life data showed shorter hospital stays and about 88% of subjects who had laparoscopic surgery recovered completely within 12 months as compared with 58% who had open surgery.[91] However, evidence for laparoscopic resections for rectal cancers is less clear.[92–94] Studies looking at the feasibility of laparoscopic surgery for rectal cancers have reported that laparoscopic resection and a fast-track program complement each other leading to better outcomes, and they can be safely implemented in a general surgical unit.[95,96]

Evidence of Enhanced Recovery After Surgery from Randomized Controlled Trials

A recent meta-analysis[97] of RCTs[98–103] has reported that subjects undergoing major open colorectal surgery and managed with a perioperative ERAS pathway had a primary hospital stay of 2.5 days less than those managed with a traditional-care pathway, and had significantly fewer postoperative complications. There were no statistically significant differences in readmission and mortality rates (**Table 4**).

EVIDENCE FROM OTHER SPECIALTIES

ERAS pathways have also shown positive outcomes, such as decreased length of stay and complications, in patients undergoing surgical procedures other than colorectal surgery, such as thoracic,[104] vascular,[105,106] orthopedics, urology,[107–110] esophageal,[111,112] pancreatic,[113–115] and liver[116,117] surgery. However, the evidence is limited and needs further evaluation in future prospective studies.

COSTS AND SAVINGS

Evidence presented for individual elements of the ERAS pathway in the perioperative period result in favorable outcomes without increasing readmission or mortality rates. Although factors, such as patients' fear or anxiety, preoperative organ dysfunction, surgical stress response, perioperative hypothermia, hypoxemia, nausea, vomiting, ileus, sleep disturbance, semi-starvation, nasogastric tubes, and drains and catheters, can delay recovery, ERAS addresses these factors by preoperative information/ psychological preparation, optimizing associated physiologic dysfunction, correcting nutritional defects, modifying alcohol abuse and smoking, epidural blockade, minimally invasive operations, maintenance of normothermia and oxygen delivery, nausea and ileus prevention, early feeding, disturbance-free sleep time, opioid sparing analgesia, and evidence-based postoperative care. Although avoiding routine bowel preparation and prolonged preoperative fasting; using intravenous fluids, drains, and nasogastric tubes; and reducing nursing time and hospital stay all decrease the overall costs, factors, such as preoperative counseling, patient and staff education, early mobilization, and perioperative nutrition, can potentially increase the health care costs in the short term. However, some studies have reported successful implementation of ERAS elements with economic benefits at no increased costs without increasing the complication or readmission rates.[2,118] The economic benefit of laparoscopic colorectal surgery, however, still remains unclear.[119] There are inconsistencies in reporting cost effectiveness,[92] though some studies have reported short-term and long-term clinical benefits, including fewer complications,[120–122] similar survival, and cure rates up to 3 years.[123] Changes in nursing tasks with reduction in postoperative nursing care per day and per stay have been reported with no increased demands on nursing time.[124,125] Although the exact savings may vary between units and health care systems, undoubtedly shortening length of stay by 2 to 3 days saves resources and decreasing complication rates by up to 50% reduces cost and suffering.

IMPLEMENTATION: DIFFICULTIES AND SOLUTIONS

The implementation of ERAS pathways, despite demonstration of advantages with regards to clinical outcomes, such as length of stay, complications, readmissions, or mortality, have been slow or have not been applied optimally in many centers.[47,126,127] Even though individual elements of ERAS pathways are based on evidence-based principles that have been successfully implemented in dedicated centers and district general hospitals,[128–132] critics argue that reported advantages in outcomes, such as shorter lengths of stay, could relate to changes in organizational structure following implementation of fast-track programs and evidence regarding recovery and follow-up should be reported in more detail in ERAS programs.[133] A study reporting improved outcomes, such as early feeding, early mobilization, and

Table 4
Summary of outcomes: evidence from six RCTs comparing eras with traditional care in patients undergoing major elective open colorectal surgery

Outcome	Studies	Participants	Statistical Method	Effect Estimate	Heterogeneity (I^2) and P Value
Length of hospital stay	6	452	Mean difference (IV, random, 95% CI)	-2.51 (-3.54, -1.47)	$I^2 = 55\%$, P<.00001
Complications	6	452	Risk ratio (M-H, random, 95% CI)	0.53 (0.41, 0.69)	$I^2 = 0\%$; P<.00001
Readmissions	6	452	Risk ratio (M-H, random, 95% CI)	0.80 (0.32, 1.98)	$I^2 = 9\%$; P = .62
Mortality	6	452	Risk ratio (M-H, random, 95% CI)	0.53 (0.09, 3.15)	$I^2 = 0\%$; P = .49

Effect estimate for experimental group (ERAS) compared with control group (traditional care). The degree of heterogeneity is proportional to the I^2 value.
Abbreviations: CI, confidence interval; IV, inverse variance; M-H, Mantel-Haenszel.
Data from Varadhan KK, Neal KR, Dejong CHC, et al. The enhanced recovery after surgery (ERAS) pathway for patients undergoing major elective open colorectal surgery: a meta-analysis of randomised controlled trials. Clin Nutr 2010. [Epub ahead of print]. DOI:10.1016/j.clnu.2010.01.004.

early return of bowel function, before and immediately after implementing the enhanced recovery program also showed that despite resulting in increased readmission rates, the total hospital stay was still lower compared with traditional care, with decreased risk for complications in colonic surgery and no change in complication rates in rectal surgery. However, implementation of ERAS protocols in a shared-practice environment creates a complementary pattern of change, which favored better outcomes for all patients, regardless of treatment by ERAS or traditional methods[134] and without comprising the workload or working environment of nursing staff.[124] Another study reported, despite incomplete implementation, ERAS protocols showed good results when compared with traditional care.[135] Successful implementation of ERAS pathways have been reported following a brief preparatory period, emphasizing the need for staff and patient education in achieving the intended goals of ERAS pathways.[124,136,137] There is also evidence to support the fact that elderly patients fare better when treated within an ERAS pathway and that age and nutritional status are not independent determinants of morbidity or mortality[16] and improved patient satisfaction and quality of life with ERAS pathways.[21,138]

Although several studies and meta-analyses over the last few years have shown that patients benefit from ERAS programs, implementing ERAS pathways across multiple institutions has remained a challenge. Despite sometimes overwhelming evidence in its favor, the acceptance of principles of ERAS has been slow among different health care systems and clinicians in many countries. A way forward seems to be to focus on identifying the pitfalls that inhibit implementation of ERAS programs, so that further developments can be made within health care infrastructures for successful delivery of ERAS pathways.[139] Improved application of ERAS pathways through staff and patient education, a multidisciplinary approach to patient care, maintaining compliance to ERAS elements, improving rehabilitation processes, benchmarking standards of care, and monitoring of performance against national and international standards are recommended to further improve resource use and health care delivery across all surgical specialties.

SUMMARY

In units where ERAS has been studied or implemented, the evidence shows marked improvements in patient care and outcome. ERAS results in substantially faster recovery of function and significantly fewer complications. Although there are no exact figures available, these improvements also represent economic benefits to the society. These improvements have been shown for patients undergoing elective colorectal surgery, and there are reports demonstrating similar improvements in many other types of surgery. Although the multimodal approach yields positive results, it is less clear which specific components are particularly important for these improvements. This matter remains to be studied. Despite the overwhelming improvements in the results, it is difficult to implement the principles of ERAS in day-to-day general surgical practice. Most units in the world cling to old and outdated traditional care principles. It is only in some select centers that implementation of ERAS has been successful. To successfully have the change of practice take place in a large number of hospitals, a structured program for the implementation of ERAS seems to be the most successful method employed so far. To secure the wide-spread use of modern care and to find ways of securing the implementation of improved-care pathways in daily surgical practice remains the main challenge for the surgical community. The evidence is already there, it is the inner will and strength to change that is missing.

REFERENCES

1. Kehlet H. Multimodal approach to control postoperative pathophysiology and rehabilitation. Br J Anaesth 1997;78:606–17.
2. King PM, Blazeby JM, Ewings P, et al. The influence of an enhanced recovery programme on clinical outcomes, costs and quality of life after surgery for colorectal cancer. Colorectal Dis 2006;8:506–13.
3. Eskicioglu C, Forbes SS, Aarts MA, et al. Enhanced recovery after surgery (ERAS) programs for patients having colorectal surgery: a meta-analysis of randomized trials. J Gastrointest Surg 2009;13:2321–9.
4. Gouvas N, Tan E, Windsor A, et al. Fast-track vs standard care in colorectal surgery: a meta-analysis update. Int J Colorectal Dis 2009;24:1119–31.
5. Walter CJ, Collin J, Dumville JC, et al. Enhanced recovery in colorectal resections: a systematic review and meta-analysis. Colorectal Dis 2009;11:344–53.
6. Fearon KC, Ljungqvist O, Von Meyenfeldt M, et al. Enhanced recovery after surgery: a consensus review of clinical care for patients undergoing colonic resection. Clin Nutr 2005;24:466–77.
7. Lassen K, Soop M, Nygren J, et al. Consensus review of optimal perioperative care in colorectal surgery: enhanced recovery after surgery (ERAS) Group recommendations. Arch Surg 2009;144:961–9.
8. Kehlet H, Mogensen T. Hospital stay of 2 days after open sigmoidectomy with a multimodal rehabilitation programme. Br J Surg 1999;86:227–30.
9. Delaney CP, Fazio VW, Senagore AJ, et al. 'Fast track' postoperative management protocol for patients with high co-morbidity undergoing complex abdominal and pelvic colorectal surgery. Br J Surg 2001;88:1533–8.

10. Nygren J, Hausel J, Kehlet H, et al. A comparison in five European centres of case mix, clinical management and outcomes following either conventional or fast-track perioperative care in colorectal surgery. Clin Nutr 2005;24:455–61.
11. Lassen K, Hannemann P, Ljungqvist O, et al. Patterns in current perioperative practice: survey of colorectal surgeons in five northern European countries. BMJ 2005;330:1420–1.
12. Hannemann P, Lassen K, Hausel J, et al. Patterns in current anaesthesiologic perioperative practice for colonic resections. A survey in 5 Northern-European countries. Acta Anaesthesiol Scand 2006;50:1152–60.
13. Maessen J, Dejong CH, Hausel J, et al. A protocol is not enough to implement an enhanced recovery programme for colorectal resection. Br J Surg 2007;94: 224–31.
14. Nygren J, Soop M, Thorell A, et al. An enhanced-recovery protocol improves outcome after colorectal resection already during the first year: a single-center experience in 168 consecutive patients. Dis Colon Rectum 2009;52:978–85.
15. Hausel J, Nygren J, Gustafsson U, et al. Enhanced recovery programs reduce complications after colorectal surgery [abstract]. Clin Nutr Suppl 2008;3(S1):26.
16. Hendry PO, Hausel J, Nygren J, et al. Determinants of outcome after colorectal resection within an enhanced recovery programme. Br J Surg 2009;96:197–205.
17. Holte K, Nielsen KG, Madsen JL, et al. Physiologic effects of bowel preparation. Dis Colon Rectum 2004;47:1397–402.
18. Lobo DN. Fluid, electrolytes and nutrition: physiological and clinical aspects. Proc Nutr Soc 2004;63:453–66.
19. Lobo DN. Fluid overload and surgical outcome: another piece in the jigsaw. Ann Surg 2009;249:186–8.
20. Arora NS, Rochester DF. Respiratory muscle strength and maximal voluntary ventilation in undernourished patients. Am Rev Respir Dis 1982;126:5–8.
21. Blazeby JM, Soulsby M, Winstone K, et al. A qualitative evaluation of patients' experiences of an enhanced recovery programme for colorectal cancer. Colorectal Dis 2009. [Epub ahead of print]. DOI:10.1111/j.1463–1318.2009.02104.x.
22. Disbrow EA, Bennett HL, Owings JT. Effect of preoperative suggestion on postoperative gastrointestinal motility. West J Med 1993;158:488–92.
23. Egbert LD, Battit GE, Welch CE, et al. Reduction of postoperative pain by encouragement and instruction of patients. A study of doctor-patient rapport. N Engl J Med 1964;270:825–7.
24. Giner M, Laviano A, Meguid MM, et al. In 1995 a correlation between malnutrition and poor outcome in critically ill patients still exists. Nutrition 1996;12: 23–9.
25. Guenaga KK, Matos D, Wille-Jørgensen P. Mechanical bowel preparation for elective colorectal surgery. Cochrane Database Syst Rev 2009;1:CD001544.
26. Jung B, Pahlman L, Nystrom PO, et al. Multicentre randomized clinical trial of mechanical bowel preparation in elective colonic resection. Br J Surg 2007; 94:689–95.
27. Klafta JM, Roizen MF. Current understanding of patients' attitudes toward and preparation for anesthesia: a review. Anesth Analg 1996;83:1314–21.
28. Mahomed NN, Liang MH, Cook EF, et al. The importance of patient expectations in predicting functional outcomes after total joint arthroplasty. J Rheumatol 2002; 29:1273–9.
29. Naber TH, Schermer T, de Bree A, et al. Prevalence of malnutrition in nonsurgical hospitalized patients and its association with disease complications. Am J Clin Nutr 1997;66:1232–9.

30. Platell C, Hall J. What is the role of mechanical bowel preparation in patients undergoing colorectal surgery? Dis Colon Rectum 1998;41:875–82 [discussion: 82–3].
31. Ram E, Sherman Y, Weil R, et al. Is mechanical bowel preparation mandatory for elective colon surgery? A prospective randomized study. Arch Surg 2005; 140:285–8.
32. Schutz T, Pirlich M. Malnutrition in the hospital: age as a special risk factor. Pflege Z 2006;59:778–9.
33. Slim K, Vicaut E, Panis Y, et al. Meta-analysis of randomized clinical trials of colorectal surgery with or without mechanical bowel preparation. Br J Surg 2004;91:1125–30.
34. Svanfeldt M, Thorell A, Hausel J, et al. Randomized clinical trial of the effect of preoperative oral carbohydrate treatment on postoperative whole-body protein and glucose kinetics. Br J Surg 2007;94:1342–50.
35. Frank SM, Fleisher LA, Breslow MJ, et al. Perioperative maintenance of normothermia reduces the incidence of morbid cardiac events. A randomized clinical trial. JAMA 1997;277:1127–34.
36. Jesus EC, Karliczek A, Matos D, et al. Prophylactic anastomotic drainage for colorectal surgery. Cochrane Database Syst Rev 2004;4:CD002100.
37. Kurz A, Sessler DI, Lenhardt R. Perioperative normothermia to reduce the incidence of surgical-wound infection and shorten hospitalization. Study of Wound Infection and Temperature Group. N Engl J Med 1996;334:1209–15.
38. Lin JH, Whelan RL, Sakellarios NE, et al. Prospective study of ambulation after open and laparoscopic colorectal resection. Surg Innov 2009;16:16–20.
39. Lobo DN, Bostock KA, Neal KR, et al. Effect of salt and water balance on recovery of gastrointestinal function after elective colonic resection: a randomised controlled trial. Lancet 2002;359:1812–8.
40. Lobo DN, Dube MG, Neal KR, et al. Peri-operative fluid and electrolyte management: a survey of consultant surgeons in the UK. Ann R Coll Surg Engl 2002;84: 156–60.
41. Nesher N, Zisman E, Wolf T, et al. Strict thermoregulation attenuates myocardial injury during coronary artery bypass graft surgery as reflected by reduced levels of cardiac-specific troponin I. Anesth Analg 2003;96:328–35.
42. Nisanevich V, Felsenstein I, Almogy G, et al. Effect of intraoperative fluid management on outcome after intra-abdominal surgery. Anesthesiology 2005; 103:25–32.
43. Schmied H, Kurz A, Sessler DI, et al. Mild hypothermia increases blood loss and transfusion requirements during total hip arthroplasty. Lancet 1996;347:289–92.
44. Scott EM, Buckland R. A systematic review of intraoperative warming to prevent postoperative complications. AORN J 2006;83:1090–104, 107–13.
45. Vlug MS, Wind J, van der Zaag E, et al. Systematic review of laparoscopic vs open colonic surgery within an enhanced recovery programme. Colorectal Dis 2009;11:335–43.
46. Zerey M, Burns JM, Kercher KW, et al. Minimally invasive management of colon cancer. Surg Innov 2006;13:5–15.
47. Hasenberg T, Rittler P, Post S, et al. A survey of perioperative therapy for elective colon resection in Germany, 2006. Chirurg 2007;78:818–26.
48. Kaska M, Grosmanova T, Havel E, et al. Preparation of patients for operation with per-oral intake on the day of the planned surgery. Rozhl Chir 2006;85:554–9.
49. Miedema BW, Johnson JO. Methods for decreasing postoperative gut dysmotility. Lancet Oncol 2003;4:365–72.

50. Moiniche S, Kehlet H, Dahl JB. A qualitative and quantitative systematic review of preemptive analgesia for postoperative pain relief: the role of timing of analgesia. Anesthesiology 2002;96:725–41.

51. Noblett SE, Watson DS, Huong H, et al. Pre-operative oral carbohydrate loading in colorectal surgery: a randomized controlled trial. Colorectal Dis 2006;8: 563–9.

52. Nygren J, Thorell A, Ljungqvist O. Preoperative oral carbohydrate nutrition: an update. Curr Opin Clin Nutr Metab Care 2001;4:255–9.

53. Walker KJ, Smith AF. Premedication for anxiety in adult day surgery. Cochrane Database Syst Rev 2009;4:CD002192.

54. Yuill KA, Richardson RA, Davidson HI, et al. The administration of an oral carbohydrate-containing fluid prior to major elective upper-gastrointestinal surgery preserves skeletal muscle mass postoperatively–a randomised clinical trial. Clin Nutr 2005;24:32–7.

55. Andersen J, Hjort-Jakobsen D, Christiansen PS, et al. Readmission rates after a planned hospital stay of 2 versus 3 days in fast-track colonic surgery. Br J Surg 2007;94:890–3.

56. Basse L, Hjort Jakobsen D, Billesbolle P, et al. A clinical pathway to accelerate recovery after colonic resection. Ann Surg 2000;232:51–7.

57. Basse L, Madsen JL, Kehlet H. Normal gastrointestinal transit after colonic resection using epidural analgesia, enforced oral nutrition and laxative. Br J Surg 2001;88:1498–500.

58. Basse L, Werner M, Kehlet H. Is urinary drainage necessary during continuous epidural analgesia after colonic resection? Reg Anesth Pain Med 2000;25: 498–501.

59. Bisgaard T, Kehlet H. Early oral feeding after elective abdominal surgery–what are the issues? Nutrition 2002;18:944–8.

60. Block BM, Liu SS, Rowlingson AJ, et al. Efficacy of postoperative epidural analgesia: a meta-analysis. JAMA 2003;290:2455–63.

61. Kehlet H, Wilmore DW. Multimodal strategies to improve surgical outcome. Am J Surg 2002;183:630–41.

62. Lassen K, Kjaeve J, Fetveit T, et al. Allowing normal food at will after major upper gastrointestinal surgery does not increase morbidity: a randomized multicenter trial. Ann Surg 2008;247:721–9.

63. Lewis SJ, Andersen HK, Thomas S. Early enteral nutrition within 24 h of intestinal surgery versus later commencement of feeding: a systematic review and meta-analysis. J Gastrointest Surg 2009;13:569–75.

64. Maessen JM, Hoff C, Jottard K, et al. To eat or not to eat: facilitating early oral intake after elective colonic surgery in the Netherlands. Clin Nutr 2009;28:29–33.

65. Marret E, Remy C, Bonnet F. Meta-analysis of epidural analgesia versus parenteral opioid analgesia after colorectal surgery. Br J Surg 2007;94:665–73.

66. Nelson R, Edwards S, Tse B. Prophylactic nasogastric decompression after abdominal surgery. Cochrane Database Syst Rev 2007;3:CD004929.

67. Taqi A, Hong X, Mistraletti G, et al. Thoracic epidural analgesia facilitates the restoration of bowel function and dietary intake in patients undergoing laparoscopic colon resection using a traditional, non-accelerated, perioperative care program. Surg Endosc 2007;21:247–52.

68. Turunen P, Carpelan-Holmstrom M, Kairaluoma P, et al. Epidural analgesia diminished pain but did not otherwise improve enhanced recovery after laparoscopic sigmoidectomy: a prospective randomized study. Surg Endosc 2009;23:31–7.

69. Urbach DR, Kennedy ED, Cohen MM. Colon and rectal anastomoses do not require routine drainage: a systematic review and meta-analysis. Ann Surg 1999;229:174–80.
70. Wald HL, Ma A, Bratzler DW, et al. Indwelling urinary catheter use in the postoperative period: analysis of the national surgical infection prevention project data. Arch Surg 2008;143:551–7.
71. Yang Z, Zheng Q, Wang Z. Meta-analysis of the need for nasogastric or nasojejunal decompression after gastrectomy for gastric cancer. Br J Surg 2008; 95:809–16.
72. Thorell A, Nygren J, Ljungqvist O. Insulin resistance: a marker of surgical stress. Curr Opin Clin Nutr Metab Care 1999;2:69–78.
73. Stratton RJ, Green CJ, Elia M. Disease-related malnutrition: an evidence-based approach to treatment. Oxford (UK): CABI Publishing; 2003.
74. Brady M, Kinn S, Stuart P. Preoperative fasting for adults to prevent perioperative complications. Cochrane Database Syst Rev 2003;4:CD004423.
75. Carlisle JB, Stevenson CA. Drugs for preventing postoperative nausea and vomiting. Cochrane Database Syst Rev 2006;3:CD004125.
76. McLeod RS, Geerts WH, Sniderman KW, et al. Subcutaneous heparin versus low-molecular-weight heparin as thromboprophylaxis in patients undergoing colorectal surgery: results of the Canadian colorectal DVT prophylaxis trial: a randomized, double-blind trial. Ann Surg 2001;233:438–44.
77. Platell C, Barwood N, Makin G. Randomized clinical trial of bowel preparation with a single phosphate enema or polyethylene glycol before elective colorectal surgery. Br J Surg 2006;93:427–33.
78. Song F, Glenny AM. Antimicrobial prophylaxis in colorectal surgery: a systematic review of randomized controlled trials. Br J Surg 1998;85:1232–41.
79. Wallenborn J, Gelbrich G, Bulst D, et al. Prevention of postoperative nausea and vomiting by metoclopramide combined with dexamethasone: randomised double blind multicentre trial. BMJ 2006;333:324–7.
80. Wille-Jorgensen P, Rasmussen MS, Andersen BR, et al. Heparins and mechanical methods for thromboprophylaxis in colorectal surgery. Cochrane Database Syst Rev 2003;4:CD001217.
81. Westergren A, Wann-Hansson C, Borgdal EB, et al. Malnutrition prevalence and precision in nutritional care differed in relation to hospital volume–a cross-sectional survey. Nutr J 2009;8:20.
82. Braga M, Ljungqvist O, Soeters P, et al. ESPEN Guidelines on Parenteral Nutrition: surgery. Clin Nutr 2009;28:378–86.
83. Weimann A, Braga M, Harsanyi L, et al. ESPEN Guidelines on Enteral Nutrition: Surgery including organ transplantation. Clin Nutr 2006;25:224–44.
84. Phillips B, BC, Sacket D, et al. Levels of evidence and grades of recommendations. Centre for evidence based medicine; University of Oxford; 2007. Available from: http://www.cebm.net/index.aspx?o=1025. Accessed January 12, 2010.
85. Braga M, Ljungqvist O, Soeters P, et al. ESPEN guidelines on parenteral nutrition: surgery. Clin Nutr 2009;28:378–86.
86. Abraham NS, Byrne CM, Young JM, et al. Meta-analysis of non-randomized comparative studies of the short-term outcomes of laparoscopic resection for colorectal cancer. ANZ J Surg 2007;77:508–16.
87. Liang Y, Li G, Chen P, et al. Laparoscopic versus open colorectal resection for cancer: a meta-analysis of results of randomized controlled trials on recurrence. Eur J Surg Oncol 2008;34:1217–24.

88. Schwenk W, Haase O, Neudecker J, et al. Short term benefits for laparoscopic colorectal resection. Cochrane Database Syst Rev 2005;3:CD003145.
89. Raymond T, Kumar S, Dastur J, et al. Case controlled study of the hospital stay and return to full activity following laparoscopic and open colorectal surgery before and after the introduction of an enhanced recovery programme. Colorectal Dis 2009. [Epub ahead of print]. DOI:10.1111/j.1463-1318.2009.01925.x.
90. Raymond TM, Dastur JK, Khot UP, et al. Hospital stay and return to full activity following laparoscopic colorectal surgery. JSLS 2008;12:143-9.
91. King PM, Blazeby JM, Ewings P, et al. Detailed evaluation of functional recovery following laparoscopic or open surgery for colorectal cancer within an enhanced recovery programme. Int J Colorectal Dis 2008;23:795-800.
92. Faiz O, Kennedy R. The cost of laparoscopic colorectal surgery. Colorectal Dis 2009;11:431-2.
93. Koopmann MC, Heise CP. Laparoscopic and minimally invasive resection of malignant colorectal disease. Surg Clin North Am 2008;88:1047-72.
94. Kienle P, Weitz J, Koch M, et al. Laparoscopic surgery for colorectal cancer. Colorectal Dis 2006;8(Suppl 3):33-6.
95. Spatz H, Zulke C, Beham A, et al. Fast-Track for laparoscopic-assisted rectum resection—what can be achieved? First results of a feasibility study. Zentralbl Chir 2006;131:383-7.
96. Scatizzi M, Kroning KC, Boddi V, et al. Fast-track surgery after laparoscopic colorectal surgery: is it feasible in a general surgery unit? Surgery 2009. [Epub ahead of print]. DOI:10.1016/j.surg.2009.09.035.
97. Varadhan KK, Neal KR, Dejong CHC, et al. The enhanced recovery after surgery (ERAS) pathway for patients undergoing major elective open colorectal surgery: a meta-analysis of randomised controlled trials. Clin Nutr 2010. [Epub ahead of print]. DOI:10.1016/j.clnu.2010.01.004.
98. Anderson AD, McNaught CE, MacFie J, et al. Randomized clinical trial of multimodal optimization and standard perioperative surgical care. Br J Surg 2003;90:1497-504.
99. Delaney CP, Zutshi M, Senagore AJ, et al. Prospective, randomized, controlled trial between a pathway of controlled rehabilitation with early ambulation and diet and traditional postoperative care after laparotomy and intestinal resection. Dis Colon Rectum 2003;46:851-9.
100. Gatt M, Anderson AD, Reddy BS, et al. Randomized clinical trial of multimodal optimization of surgical care in patients undergoing major colonic resection. Br J Surg 2005;92:1354-62.
101. Khoo CK, Vickery CJ, Forsyth N, et al. A prospective randomized controlled trial of multimodal perioperative management protocol in patients undergoing elective colorectal resection for cancer. Ann Surg 2007;245:867-72.
102. Muller S, Zalunardo MP, Hubner M, et al. A fast-track program reduces complications and length of hospital stay after open colonic surgery. Gastroenterology 2009;136:842-7.
103. Serclová Z, Dytrych P, Marvan J, et al. Fast-track in open intestinal surgery: prospective randomized study. (Clinical Trials Gov Identifier no. NCT00123456). Clin Nutr 2009;28:618-24.
104. McKenna RJ Jr, Mahtabifard A, Pickens A, et al. Fast-tracking after video-assisted thoracoscopic surgery lobectomy, segmentectomy, and pneumonectomy. Ann Thorac Surg 2007;84:1663-7 [discussion: 7-8].
105. Muehling B, Schelzig H, Steffen P, et al. A prospective randomized trial comparing traditional and fast-track patient care in elective open infrarenal aneurysm repair. World J Surg 2009;33:577-85.

106. Murphy MA, Richards T, Atkinson C, et al. Fast track open aortic surgery: reduced post operative stay with a goal directed pathway. Eur J Vasc Endovasc Surg 2007;34:274–8.
107. Arumainayagam N, McGrath J, Jefferson KP, et al. Introduction of an enhanced recovery protocol for radical cystectomy. BJU Int 2008;101:698–701.
108. Chughtai B, Abraham C, Finn D, et al. Fast track open partial nephrectomy: reduced postoperative length of stay with a goal-directed pathway does not compromise outcome. Adv Urol 2008:507543.
109. Gralla O, Haas F, Knoll N, et al. Fast-track surgery in laparoscopic radical prostatectomy: basic principles. World J Urol 2007;25:185–91.
110. Maffezzini M, Campodonico F, Canepa G, et al. Current perioperative management of radical cystectomy with intestinal urinary reconstruction for muscle-invasive bladder cancer and reduction of the incidence of postoperative ileus. Surg Oncol 2008;17:41–8.
111. Jiang K, Cheng L, Wang JJ, et al. Fast track clinical pathway implications in esophagogastrectomy. World J Gastroenterol 2009;15:496–501.
112. Low DE. Evolution in perioperative management of patients undergoing oesophagectomy. Br J Surg 2007;94:655–6.
113. Balzano G, Zerbi A, Braga M, et al. Fast-track recovery programme after pancreatico- duodenectomy reduces delayed gastric emptying. Br J Surg 2008; 95:1387–93.
114. Berberat PO, Ingold H, Gulbinas A, et al. Fast track–different implications in pancreatic surgery. J Gastrointest Surg 2007;11:880–7.
115. Kennedy EP, Rosato EL, Sauter PK, et al. Initiation of a critical pathway for pancreaticoduodenectomy at an academic institution–the first step in multi-disciplinary team building. J Am Coll Surg 2007;204:917–23 [discussion: 923–4].
116. MacKay G, O'Dwyer PJ. Early discharge following liver resection for colorectal metastases. Scott Med J 2008;53:22–4.
117. van Dam RM, Hendry PO, Coolsen MM, et al. Initial experience with a multimodal enhanced recovery programme in patients undergoing liver resection. Br J Surg 2008;95:969–75.
118. Kariv Y, Delaney CP, Senagore AJ, et al. Clinical outcomes and cost analysis of a "fast track" postoperative care pathway for ileal pouch-anal anastomosis: a case control study. Dis Colon Rectum 2007;50:137–46.
119. Khan S, Gatt M, MacFie J. Enhanced recovery programmes and colorectal surgery: does the laparoscope confer additional advantages? Colorectal Dis 2009;11:902–8.
120. Delaney CP, Chang E, Senagore AJ, et al. Clinical outcomes and resource utilization associated with laparoscopic and open colectomy using a large national database. Ann Surg 2008;247:819–24.
121. Aly EH. Laparoscopic colorectal surgery: summary of the current evidence. Ann R Coll Surg Engl 2009;91:541–4.
122. Kaido T. Current evidence supporting indications for laparoscopic surgery in colorectal cancer. Hepatogastroenterology 2008;55:438–41.
123. Murray A, Lourenco T, de Verteuil R, et al. Clinical effectiveness and cost-effectiveness of laparoscopic surgery for colorectal cancer: systematic reviews and economic evaluation. Health Technol Assess 2006;10:1–141.
124. Sjetne IS, Krogstad U, Odegard S, et al. Improving quality by introducing enhanced recovery after surgery in a gynaecological department: consequences for ward nursing practice. Qual Saf Health Care 2009;18:236–40.

125. Jakobsen DH, Sonne E, Andreasen J, et al. Convalescence after colonic surgery with fast-track vs conventional care. Colorectal Dis 2006;8:683–7.
126. Kehlet H, Wilmore DW. Evidence-based surgical care and the evolution of fast-track surgery. Ann Surg 2008;248:189–98.
127. Kehlet H, Buchler MW, Beart RW Jr, et al. Care after colonic operation–is it evidence-based? Results from a multinational survey in Europe and the United States. J Am Coll Surg 2006;202:45–54.
128. Hammer J, Harling H, Wille-Jorgensen P. Implementation of the scientific evidence into daily practice–example from fast-track colonic cancer surgery. Colorectal Dis 2008;10:593–8.
129. Jottard K, Hoff C, Maessen J, et al. Life and death of the nasogastric tube in elective colonic surgery in the Netherlands. Clin Nutr 2009;28:26–8.
130. Ionescu D, Iancu C, Ion D, et al. Implementing fast-track protocol for colorectal surgery: a prospective randomized clinical trial. World J Surg 2009;33:2433–8.
131. Bosio RM, Smith BM, Aybar PS, et al. Implementation of laparoscopic colectomy with fast-track care in an academic medical center: benefits of a fully ascended learning curve and specialty expertise. Am J Surg 2007;193:413–5 [discussion: 5–6].
132. Jottard KJ, van Berlo C, Jeuken L, et al. Changes in outcome during implementation of a fast-track colonic surgery project in a university-affiliated general teaching hospital: advantages reached with ERAS (Enhanced Recovery After Surgery project) over a 1-year period. Dig Surg 2008;25:335–8.
133. Maessen JM, Dejong CH, Kessels AG, et al. Length of stay: an inappropriate readout of the success of enhanced recovery programs. World J Surg 2008; 32:971–5.
134. Sailhamer EA, Sokal SM, Chang Y, et al. Environmental impact of accelerated clinical care in a high-volume center. Surgery 2007;142:343–9.
135. Polle SW, Wind J, Fuhring JW, et al. Implementation of a fast-track perioperative care program: what are the difficulties? Dig Surg 2007;24:441–9.
136. Mohn AC, Bernardshaw SV, Ristesund SM, et al. Enhanced recovery after colorectal surgery. Results from a prospective observational two-centre study. Scand J Surg 2009;98:155–9.
137. Scharfenberg M, Raue W, Junghans T, et al. Fast-track rehabilitation after colonic surgery in elderly patients–is it feasible? Int J Colorectal Dis 2007;22: 1469–74.
138. Khan S, Wilson T, Ahmed J, et al. Quality of life and patient satisfaction with enhanced recovery protocols. Colorectal Dis 2009. [Epub ahead of print]. DOI:10.1111/j.1463-1318.2009.01997.x.
139. Kehlet H. Multimodal approach to postoperative recovery. Curr Opin Crit Care 2009;15:355–8.

Can We Protect the Gut in Critical Illness? The Role of Growth Factors and Other Novel Approaches

Jessica A. Dominguez, PhD[a],*, Craig M. Coopersmith, MD[b]

KEYWORDS

• Critical illness • Intestine • Growth factors

For more than two decades, the gut has been hypothesized as the "motor" of the systemic inflammatory response syndrome. As critical care research has evolved, many studies have defined how the gut plays a role in the origin and propagation of critical illness. During shock, intestinal hypoperfusion followed by reperfusion leads to production of proinflammatory mediators that can amplify the systemic inflammatory response.[1] Interactions between host and bacterial pathogens in the intestine contribute to gut-derived sepsis.[2] Intestinal permeability in critical illness, as a result of compromised epithelial tight junctions, leads to persistent activation of systemic inflammation.[3–5] Toxic gut-derived substances enter the mesenteric lymph, leading to lung damage, and distant organ injury can be prevented by ligating the mesenteric lymph duct in hemorrhagic shock.[6] Intestinal epithelial apoptosis is elevated after sepsis, and prevention of sepsis-induced intestinal apoptosis by overexpression of the antiapoptotic protein, Bcl-2, improves survival in several animal models of sepsis.[7,8]

Because perturbations to the intestinal epithelium can cause distant organ damage and development of multiple organ dysfunction syndrome, identifying ways to preserve intestinal integrity may be of paramount importance in the treatment of critical illness. Growth factors have emerged as potential tools for modulation of intestinal inflammation and repair, playing important roles in cellular proliferation, differentiation,

This work was supported by from the National Institutes of Health (GM66202, GM072808, and F32 GM082008) and the Shock Society Research Fellowship for Early Career Investigators.
[a] Department of Anesthesiology, University of Colorado Denver School of Medicine, 12700 East 19th Avenue, Campus Box 8602, Aurora, CO 80045, USA
[b] Department of Surgery, Emory University School of Medicine, 101 Woodruff Circle, Suite WMB 5101, Atlanta, GA 30322, USA
* Corresponding author.
E-mail address: Jessica.dominguez@ucdenver.edu

migration, and survival. This review examines the involvement of growth factors and other peptides in intestinal mucosal repair during critical illness and their potential use as therapeutic targets.

MUCOSAL REPAIR IN THE GASTROINTESTINAL TRACT

The mucosal lining of the gastrointestinal tract represents the largest body surface in contact with the outside world (approximately 300 m^2, approximately the area of a tennis court). The intestinal epithelium consists of a single layer of columnar epithelial cells that are constantly renewed from multipotent stem cells originating in the crypts of Lieberkühn. These stem cells give rise to four major epithelial lineages: absorptive enterocytes, goblet cells, enteroendocrine cells, and Paneth cells.[9] Over the course of a 3- to 5-day lifespan, enterocytes, goblet cells, and enteroendocrine cells migrate upward along the crypt-villus axis, where they differentiate and ultimately die of apoptosis or are exfoliated whole into the lumen.[10] In contrast, Paneth cells migrate downward over the course of 5 to 8 days to the crypt base where they reside for approximately 3 weeks. Each epithelial cell is in intimate contact with its neighbors, and the integrity of the epithelium is maintained by apical junctional complexes.[11] Tight junctions are the most apical components of the complex and create a dynamic barrier to the paracellular movement of water, solutes, and immune cells.[4,12]

Although minor breaches in epithelial integrity occur daily due to mechanical strain associated with intestinal motility and physiologic digestive trauma, more extensive disruption of epithelial continuity can result from bacterial invasion, chemical injury, or tissue destruction due to ischemic, septic, and inflammatory enteropathies.[13] Rapid resealing of the intestinal barrier is essential to prevent systemic penetration of toxins, immunogens, and other factors that can lead to activation of the systemic inflammatory response. The gastrointestinal tract uses at least 3 distinct mechanisms to reestablish epithelial continuity (**Fig. 1**).[14,15] Within minutes after injury, epithelial cells bordering the zone of injury migrate into the wound to cover the denuded area. During this process, termed *epithelial restitution*, epithelial cells adjacent to the injury undergo a striking change in cell shape and phenotype. Instead of their normal columnar shape, the cells flatten and adopt a squamoid appearance, followed by extension of lammelipodia. In addition, the cells undergo brush border and junctional disassembly and become polarized along the leading edge/trailing edge axis. After the wound is

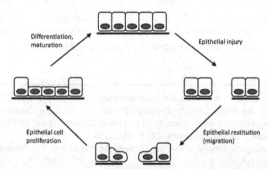

Differentiation, maturation

Epithelial injury

Epithelial cell proliferation

Epithelial restitution (migration)

Fig. 1. A simplified model of epithelial injury and restitution. After epithelial injury, cells depolarize, dedifferentiate, and migrate to cover the denuded area (restitution). Once the epithelial defect is sealed, epithelial cell proliferation is stimulated to replace the cell pool. Epithelial cells then differentiate and mature to become an intact epithelial layer again.

sealed, the cells reorganize their cytoskeleton and redifferentiate into mature entero-cytes. Epithelial cell proliferation is also stimulated to restore the functional capacity of the mucosa. Finally, undifferentiated epithelial cells undergo maturation and differen-tiation to maintain normal mucosal epithelial function. When an epithelial defect is large, stimulation of cell proliferation is crucial for restoration of normal mucosal archi-tecture. If a lesion is deep or penetrating, additional repair mechanisms are required, such as angiogenesis and deposition of extracellular matrix components to form gran-ulation tissue.

REGULATION OF INTESTINAL EPITHELIAL REPAIR BY GROWTH FACTORS

Many growth factors regulate the process of epithelial repair (**Fig. 2**).[13,16] Growth factors control a variety of activities, including stimulation of proliferation and migra-tion, cell differentiation, and acceleration of angiogenesis and extracellular matrix remodeling as well as promotion of epithelial mucosal repair.[13,16] These factors can be derived from the luminal environment as the result of intrinsic secretions from epithelial cells, or they can be produced by a variety of mucosal and submucosal cells.[13] Myofibroblasts beneath a mucosal injury secrete hepatocyte growth factor (HGF) and keratinocyte growth factor (KGF), both of which stimulate migration and proliferation of epithelial cells.[13] Neutrophils also release HGF.[17] Platelets also release growth factors in response to tissue injury, including epidermal growth factor (EGF),[18] insulin-like growth factor 1 (IGF-1),[19] and HGF.[20] These growth factors interact predominantly with receptors on the basolateral membrane of epithelial cells. In contrast, other growth factors, including intestinal trefoil factor (ITF) and glucagon-like peptide 2 (GLP-2), are secreted into the lumen and act primarily at the apical surface of epithelial cells. EGF can also be secreted into the lumen and act on the apical surface. Although a complete understanding of the complex interrelationships and redundancy of growth factors in epithelial repair remains to be determined, several studies have shed light on how these peptides protect the intestine during injury.

Epidermal Growth Factor

EGF is a potent 53 amino acid cytoprotective peptide that exhibits trophic and healing effects on the intestinal mucosa.[21,22] As a mitogen, EGF is involved with the regulation

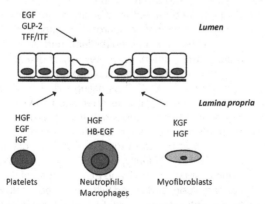

Fig. 2. Several growth factors are involved in preventing or enhancing intestinal epithelial repair.

of cellular proliferation, survival, and migration. Under basal conditions, the EGF signaling pathway is crucial for intestinal epithelial proliferation and cell survival.[23] EGF receptor (EGF-R)–deficient mice die early in postnatal life and exhibit severe defects in intestinal morphology, including fewer and shorter villi.[24] Activation of EGF-R after binding of EGF in the intestine can lead to increased blood flow,[25] increased cell survival,[26,27] decreased inflammation,[28] and improved barrier function.[29,30]

There is significantly more preclinical data on the use of EGF in adult critical illness than on other growth factors. Circulating EGF levels are decreased whereas intestinal EGF and EGF-R levels are increased after cecal ligation and puncture (CLP), a preclinical model of peritonitis-induced sepsis.[31] Animals subjected to CLP have increased sepsis-induced apoptosis, and this is associated with increased expression of BH3 interacting domain death agonist (Bid), fas-associated death domain (FADD), and p21. Apoptosis is normalized to sham levels in mice treated with exogenous EGF after the onset of sepsis, as are the levels of Bid, FADD, and p21. Septic mice also have decreased intestinal proliferation and villus length, whereas giving exogenous EGF after the onset of sepsis restores proliferation to levels seen in sham animals and nearly normalizes villus length. Giving exogenous EGF after CLP results in a 2-fold improvement in survival in septic mice.

Because EGF can have several extraintestinal effects, it was unclear whether or not the benefits conferred by exogenous EGF were enterocyte-specific. Therefore, similar experiments were performed using transgenic mice with enterocyte-specific overexpression of EGF.[30] Intestine-specific EGF overexpression is sufficient to prevent sepsis-induced decreases in intestinal proliferation and villus length and sepsis-induced increases in gut epithelial apoptosis. Furthermore, intestinal permeability is markedly increased after CLP in wild-type mice but permeability is normalized to sham levels in septic transgenic mice that overexpress EGF. This change in barrier function is associated with normalization of claudin-2 expression and localization in transgenic mice that overexpress EGF in their intestinal epithelium. Enterocyte-specific overexpression of EGF confers a marked improvement in survival in CLP-induced sepsis, suggesting the protective effects of systemic EGF in septic peritonitis are mediated in a gut-specific fashion.

In addition to improving survival in CLP, systemic administration of EGF has been demonstrated as beneficial in other models of adult critical illness. Specifically, exogenous EGF reduces intestinal injury and improves host survival in animal models of ischemia-reperfusion injury[32,33] and thermal injury.[34]

Several lines of evidence have demonstrated an important role for EGF in intestinal repair as well. In a neonatal rat model of necrotizing enterocolitis (NEC), EGF-R is significantly up-regulated in the intestinal epithelium, and supplementation of milk formula with EGF decreases the incidence and severity of disease.[35] This protection is associated with decreased intestinal epithelial apoptosis and restoration of intestinal barrier function.[27,29] The EGF/EGF-R signaling axis has also been shown to play a critical role in the adaptive response after short bowel resection because administration of exogenous EGF or enterocyte-specific overexpression of EGF enhances the adaptive response after short bowel resection.[36,37] Alternatively, this adaptive response is severely impaired in mice that lack functional EGF-R or after pharmacologic inhibition of EGF-R.[38] Finally, in patients with peptic ulcer disease, salivary levels of EGF are significantly reduced, and EGF-R expression is 75-fold higher in rats with chemically induced ulcers compared with untreated controls.[39] Patients with peptic ulcer disease treated intravenously with EGF also have improved ulcer healing compared with patients treated with cetraxate hydrochloride.[40]

Exogenous EGF seems an attractive candidate for clinical trials in critically ill patients. EGF and EGF-R have been targeted for therapeutic use in many diseases, and a federal government registration of clinical trials lists more than 200 trials involving or targeting EGF or EGF-R.[41] Although many of these trials target extraintestinal effects of EGF, beneficial effects in the gut have been reported in clinical trials with EGF. For instance, in patients with ulcerative colitis, treatment with EGF-containing enemas significantly improved scoring of disease activity, sigmoidoscopic findings, and histologic grading of injury when compared with placebo.[42] Similarly, a prospective, randomized trial with recombinant EGF in a small group of premature neonates with evidence of NEC demonstrated improved intestinal repair as determined by rectal biopsy specimens.[43] No toxicities were reported after EGF administration to these infants. Based on the benefits of EGF in preclinical trials and its apparent safety when used for short-term therapy in patients, EGF treatment may represent a novel therapeutic in critical illness.

Growth Hormone and Insulin-like Growth Factor 1

Critical illness alters the body's metabolic rate, and a prolonged hypercatabolic state is associated with increased morbidity and mortality.[44] Critical illness is also often associated with alterations in the circulating concentrations or a diminished responsiveness of tissues to anabolic proteins, such as IGF-1 and growth hormone (GH).[45]

GH is a 22-kDa anabolic protein that can antagonize some of the deleterious effects of hypercatabolism.[46] In critically ill patients, the circulating concentration of GH is markedly elevated. Despite this, there is paradoxic GH resistance, in which GH fails to stimulate IGF-1 synthesis in the liver. This has been demonstrated in preclinical trials in sheep that were injected with endotoxin[47] as well as in septic patients who were given exogenous GH but failed to increase circulating IGF-1 levels to the same extent as in controls.[48]

The receptor for GH is expressed throughout the intestine, which suggests that GH may act to promote epithelial repair during intestinal injury.[49] The response to GH in the intestine under basal and pathophysiologic conditions, however, is incompletely understood. Potent trophic effects of GH have been demonstrated in the intestine of unmanipulated transgenic mice that overexpress GH.[50] When these transgenic mice are subjected to dextran sodium sulfate (DSS)–induced colitis, they exhibit increased crypt cell proliferation resulting in improved intestinal structure.[51] Studies examining GH in animal models of short bowel syndrome have shown conflicting results with varying effects on mucosal mass.[52,53] Furthermore, a rat total parenteral nutrition model failed to demonstrate a trophic effect of GH on the intestine despite normalized body weight gain and increased plasma IGF-1 levels.[54,55] Similarly, rats given GH after severe thermal injury have improved villus morphology compared with controls, but this effect is not mediated by increased crypt cell proliferation or inhibition of epithelial apoptosis.[56]

Critical illness decreases circulating levels of IGF-1.[57] IGF-1 is a small polypeptide (70 amino acids) with considerable homology to insulin. The primary biologic effect of IGF-1 is to stimulate cellular growth and differentiation.[58,59] Several studies have demonstrated that IGF-1 has beneficial effects on intestinal homeostasis, and specific receptors for IGF-1 are present in the gastrointestinal tract of humans and animals. Under normal conditions, transgenic mice that overexpress IGF-1 exhibit increased crypt cell mitosis and increased growth of the small intestine.[60] In rats subjected to small bowel resection, administration of IGF-1 augments compensatory mucosal hyperplasia and epithelial restitution.[61] Furthermore, IGF-1 administration decreases bacterial translocation after severe thermal injury by maintaining intestinal integrity.[62,63] In addition to its effects on intestinal proliferation, IGF-1 has been shown to attenuate intestinal epithelial apoptosis in a murine model of NEC[64] and in vitro after H_2O_2-induced injury.[65]

GH and IGF-1 have been used in clinical trials. GH increased morbidity and mortality in critically ill patients in a large prospective, randomized trial.[66] Although GH has recently been hypothesized to be of potential benefit in refractory critical illness,[67] its usefulness in this setting is not proved. Long-term GH may be of benefit in patients recovering from critical illness as opposed to patients who are acutely critically ill. A recent prospective, randomized trial of long-term GH in severely burned children with greater than 40% body surface burn showed improved growth and lean body mass 2 years after the initial insult.[68] GH was initiated, however, after hospital discharge in this study, so the children were no longer critically ill by the time GH was initiated.

Therapeutic use of IGF-1 has been has not been possible because of adverse side effects, such as hypoglycemia, electrolyte imbalances, and cardiac arrest.[69,70] When IGF-1 is bound to its principle binding protein (IGFBP-3), however, it has been shown safe and efficacious in humans.[71-74] Although IGF-1/IGFBP-3 is expected to have extraintestinal effects, limited preclinical data suggest it also has beneficial effects on gut integrity. In a rat model of severe thermal injury, intravenous administration of IGF-1 in combination with IGFBP-3 stimulated small intestinal epithelial proliferation and increased villus length, crypt depth, and cell number. In addition, IGF-1/IGFBP-3 significantly decreased burn-induced intestinal epithelial apoptosis.[75] These data suggest that IGF-1/IGFBP-3 may be a potential therapeutic agent to improve intestinal integrity in critically ill patients.

Keratinocyte Growth Factor

KGF is a member of the fibroblast growth factor family that stimulates growth and differentiation of epithelial cells in the gastrointestinal tract, lung, and kidney.[76] The receptor for KGF has been found exclusively in the intestinal epithelium, suggesting that KGF acts in a paracrine manner to stimulate epithelial repair in the gut. KGF expression is markedly increased in the mucosa and submucosa of patients with inflammatory bowel disease, and KGF overexpression correlates with the degree of inflammation.[77] The fact that KGF is up-regulated after intestinal injury suggests it plays an important role in normal tissue repair. Administration of KGF to unmanipulated rats causes a marked increase in epithelial proliferation as well as a selective induction of mucin-producing goblet cells throughout the gastrointestinal tract.[78] This induction is associated with increased expression of ITFs, which also play a role in epithelial repair (discussed later). Intraperitoneal administration of KGF also reduces the extent of intestinal injury in several animal models of colitis[79] whereas KGF knockout mice subjected to DSS-induced colitis exhibit more severe colonic inflammation and delayed tissue repair than wild-type mice subjected to the same insult.[80] Exogenous KGF also promotes cell survival, because mice subjected given total parenteral nutrition exhibit decreased apoptosis and increased expression of antiapoptotic Bcl-2 proteins.[81]

Chemotherapy and irradiation can compromise epithelial integrity by rapidly killing dividing cells in the mucosa, thereby impairing normal epithelial cell renewal. These treatments are often associated with mucositis, a condition characterized by mucosal atrophy, ulceration, barrier dysfunction, and infection.[82] KGF has been successfully used as a pretreatment in animal models of gastrointestinal injury induced by radiation,[83,84] chemotherapy,[84] or a combination of both.[84] In these models, KGF increases intestinal epithelial cell survival and mucosal thickness, which is associated with decreased mortality. KGF does not effect the growth rate of epithelial tumors, suggesting it may be a good therapeutic agent to prevent intestinal damage in patients receiving cancer therapy.[84] In contrast, intravenous administration of recombinant KGF failed to induce remission in a phase II study of patients with active ulcerative colitis[85] although the dose of KGF may have been too low for any beneficial effect to be seen. The effects of KGF in critical illness are unknown.

Hepatocyte Growth Factor

HGF is a mesenchymal-derived pleiotropic protein that regulates cell proliferation, cell survival, motility, morphogenesis, anti-inflammation, and angiogenesis in a variety of cells, including gastrointestinal epithelial cells.[86,87] HGF has been shown to accelerate epithelial remodeling after injury by stimulating intestinal epithelial proliferation.[88] Administration of HGF increases mucosal mass and enhances intestinal substrate absorption in rats after small bowel resection.[89] Similarly, HGF stimulates intestinal proliferation leading to preserved villus structure in an animal model of severe thermal injury.[90] The effect of HGF on apoptosis is more variable. HGF administration inhibits intestinal epithelial apoptosis during ischemia-reperfusion injury[91] but has no effect on burn-induced intestinal apoptosis.[90]

Several studies have demonstrated that HGF promotes colonic mucosal repair in animal models of colitis. The mechanisms underlying protection vary, however, depending on the model and route of HGF treatment. In rats subjected to DSS-induced colitis, continuous intraperitoneal administration of recombinant human HGF reduces colitis-associated weight loss, colonic shortening, and improved colonic erosions, and this is associated with enhanced epithelial regeneration and cellular proliferation.[92] Similarly, daily intravenous administration of recombinant human HGF to rats with trinitrobenzene sulfonic acid-induced colitis causes a significant reduction in colonic ulcer coverage and colonic shortening, and this is associated with increased epithelial proliferation and decreased inflammatory cell infiltrate in the inflamed colon.[93] The improvements noted with intraperitoneal administration of recombinant human HGF in these models are associated with inhibition of intestinal epithelial apoptosis rather than stimulation of proliferation.[94] Several studies have reported that colitis can also be ameliorated when adenoviral-mediated, liposome-formulated, or naked HGF gene is administered intrarectally, intramuscularly, or intravenously.[95–98] A potential roadblock to using HGF in clinical trials is the observation that it may be a carcinogen because transgenic mouse strains that overexpress HGF exhibit increased rates of benign and malignant liver and mammary gland tumors.[99] The benefits or risks of short-term use of HGF in critically ill patients remain to be determined.

Heparin-Binding Epidermal Growth Factor-like Growth Factor

Heparin-binding EGF-like growth factor (HB-EGF) was first identified as a 22-kDa glycoprotein in the conditioned medium of cultured human macrophages.[100] A member of the EGF family, HB-EGF is a potent mitogen for a number of cell types, including epithelial cells, fibroblasts, smooth muscle cells, keratinocytes, and renal tubule cells.[101] Expression of endogenous HB-EGF is significantly increased in response to tissue damage, hypoxia, and oxidative stress and during wound healing and regeneration.[102] In cell culture, HB-EGF has been shown to protect intestinal epithelial cells from proinflammatory cytokine-induced apoptosis.[103] Pretreatment of intestinal epithelial cells with HB-EGF in vitro leads to decreased necrosis, preserved cytoskeletal structure, higher adenosine triphosphate levels, and improved proliferative capacity during recovery from hypoxia.[104] HB-EGF decreases the generation of reactive oxygen species in intestinal epithelial cells after ischemia-reperfusion injury.[105] HB-EGF also preserves the crypt proliferative response and decreases bacterial translocation across intestinal epithelial cell monolayers after ischemia-reperfusion injury, indicating preservation of epithelial integrity.[106]

HB-EGF has also been shown to protect the intestine in vivo. In a neonatal rat model of NEC, HB-EGF treatment caused increased intestinal proliferation and migration as well as preservation of intestinal epithelial barrier function when compared with untreated animals.[107] Furthermore, in a neonatal hemorrhagic shock model, HB-EGF treatment resulted in increased intestinal blood flow and microcirculatory flow to levels greater than basal preshock levels.[108] Although these findings are encouraging, the mechanisms for the beneficial effects of HB-EGF remain to be elucidated and its effects in adult models of critical illness have yet to be determined.

Glucagon-like Peptide 2

GLP-2 is a 33 amino acid peptide that is secreted from intestinal endocrine cells in response to nutrient ingestion, which acts as a potent growth factor for the small intestinal epithelium and, to a lesser extent, the large intestinal epithelium.[109] GLP-2 administration significantly improves morbidity and enhances epithelial repair in a diverse number of intestinal injury models, including small bowel resection,[110,111] colitis,[112,113] and enteritis.[114] The protective effects of GLP-2 are thought due to its ability to stimulate crypt cell proliferation, prevent epithelial apoptosis, enhance epithelial barrier function, and reduce intestinal permeability.[115–117]

Administration of GLP-2 or a degradation-resistant analog, h[Gly2]GLP-2, has been shown to attenuate intestinal injury in a number of preclinical models of acute disease, including necrotizing pancreatitis,[117] burn injury,[118] and ischemia-reperfusion injury.[119] In addition, it has been shown beneficial in inflammatory bowel disease.[112,114,120] Mice treated with h[Gly2]GLP-2 have preserved mucosal integrity with an increase in intestinal mass as a result of increased proliferation in DSS-induced colitis.[120] Additionally, in a murine model of indomethacin-induced enteritis, h[Gly2]GLP-2 not only stimulated proliferation but also reduced intestinal epithelial apoptosis.[114] Treatment was also associated with decreased mucosal cytokine expression, decreased myeloperoxidase activity, and a marked diminution in bacterial translocation.[114] The trophic and antiapoptotic activities of GLP-2 have also been demonstrated in rodents and pigs after withdrawal of enteral nutrition where GLP-2 infusion prevents the development of mucosal atrophy, reduces proteolysis, and decreases crypt cell apoptosis in the small intestine.[121,122]

In contrast to the significant amount of evidence supporting the use of GLP-2 in preclinical models of gut injury, limited information is available about its safety and efficacy in humans. In a small pilot study, patients with intestinal failure secondary to short bowel syndrome treated with GLP-2 had improved nutrient absorption, increased body weight, and delayed gastric emptying.[123] Further clinical evaluation of GLP-2 in humans is needed to determine if GLP-2 is effective in reducing intestinal injury or enhancing gut repair in critically ill patients.

Intestinal Trefoil Factor

The trefoil factor family (TFF) is a group of small protease-resistant peptides that are expressed in mucus-secreting epithelial cells, especially in the gastrointestinal tract. To date, 3 mammalian TFF members have been identified: TFF1, expressed by surface and pit mucus cells in the stomach; TFF2, expressed by mucus neck and glandular mucus cells of the stomach and Brunner glands of the proximal duodenum; and TFF3 (also called ITF), expressed by goblet cells of the intestine and colon.[124]

The trefoil factors have been shown to play an important role in the protection and repair of the gastrointestinal mucosa. Oral administration of TFF2 protects against ethanol-, indomethacin-, and aspirin-induced gastric injury in rats[125,126] and accelerates healing and reduces inflammation in a rat model of inflammatory bowel disease.[127] ITF also promotes epithelial cell migration and inhibits intestinal epithelial apoptosis.[128,129] Mice deficient in ITF are extremely sensitive to mucosal injury and fail to undergo any epithelial repair.[130] Increased ITF expression has been observed in proximity to sites of injury in the gastrointestinal tract, including peptic ulcers and active inflammatory bowel disease. Oral and subcutaneous administration of ITF has also been shown to protect the intestinal epithelium from a variety of insults, including ethanol, nonsteroidal anti-inflammatory drugs, and restraint stress. In addition, administration of ITF ameliorates the severity of intestinal injury in a rat model of NEC.[131] Furthermore, ITF has been shown effective in prevention and healing of acute DSS-induced colitis.[132] ITF also plays a role in protection against and recovery from intestinal mucositis induced by radiation and chemotherapy.[133] Finally, oral administration of TFF2 or ITF has been shown to significantly reduce mucosal lesions after severe thermal injury.[134,135] These studies show the trefoil factors are important regulators of intestinal epithelial repair in preclinical studies but these have not been translated into clinical findings at the bedside.

SYNERGISM BETWEEN GROWTH FACTORS

There is some evidence that growth factors may act synergistically to prevent gut injury. When given in isolation, EGF and GH-releasing peptide (GHRP)-6 have beneficial effects in animal models of intestinal injury and repair. This effect is additive, however, when EGF and GHRP-6 are given together in an ischemia-reperfusion injury model.[136] In addition, combining glutamine with GH, IGF-1, or EGF has been demonstrated to have additive or synergistic effects on intestinal growth and adaptation.[137–140] Whether or not a combination of growth factors (listed previously) will be more effective than a single growth factor in isolation in critical illness has yet to be determined.

SUMMARY

In critical illness, the gut functions as the motor of the systemic inflammatory response, and maintaining gut barrier function may be a key to preventing multiple organ dysfunction syndrome. Growth factors have been shown to play a central role in protecting the gut against injury under basal conditions and in chronic disease, and increasing evidence suggests they may play a role in acute critical illness as well. Although many of the agents (described previously) have potential therapeutic benefits, EGF is the best studied and may be the most attractive candidate for clinical trials. A synergistic approach combining growth factors may also have significant usefulness. A more complete understanding of the mechanisms through which growth factors protect the gut is needed, as are strategies for translating preclinical findings to the bedside.

REFERENCES

1. Hassoun HT, Kone BC, Mercer DW, et al. Post-injury multiple organ failure: the role of the gut. Shock 2001;15:1–10.

558 Dominguez & Coopersmith

2. Alverdy JC, Laughlin RS, Wu L. Influence of the critically ill state on host-pathogen interactions within the intestine: gut-derived sepsis redefined. Crit Care Med 2003;31:598–607.
3. Fink MP. Intestinal epithelial hyperpermeability: update on the pathogenesis of gut mucosal barrier dysfunction in critical illness. Curr Opin Crit Care 2003;9: 143–51.
4. Han X, Fink MP, Yang R, et al. Increased iNOS activity is essential for intestinal epithelial tight junction dysfunction in endotoxemic mice. Shock 2004;21:261–70.
5. Fink MP, Delude RL. Epithelial barrier dysfunction: a unifying theme to explain the pathogenesis of multiple organ dysfunction at the cellular level. Crit Care Clin 2005;21:177–96.
6. Deitch EA, Xu D, Kaise VL. Role of the gut in the development of injury- and shock induced SIRS and MODS: the gut-lymph hypothesis, a review. Front Biosci 2006;11:520–8.
7. Coopersmith CM, Stromberg PE, Dunne WM, et al. Inhibition of intestinal epithelial apoptosis and survival in a murine model of pneumonia-induced sepsis. JAMA 2002;287:1716–21.
8. Coopersmith CM, Chang KC, Swanson PE, et al. Overexpression of Bcl-2 in the intestinal epithelium improves survival in septic mice. Crit Care Med 2002;30: 195–201.
9. Cheng H, Leblond CP. Origin, differentiation and renewal of the four main epithelial cell types in the mouse small intestine. V. Unitarian theory of the origin of the four epithelial cell types. Am J Anat 1974;141:537–61.
10. Hall PA, Coates PJ, Ansari B, et al. Regulation of cell number in the mammalian gastrointestinal tract: the importance of apoptosis. J Cell Sci 1994;107(Pt 12): 3569–77.
11. Utech M, Bruwer M, Nusrat A. Tight junctions and cell-cell interactions. Methods Mol Biol 2006;341:185–95.
12. Johnson LG. Applications of imaging techniques to studies of epithelial tight junctions. Adv Drug Deliv Rev 2005;57:111–21.
13. Mammen JMVM, Matthews JBM. Mucosal repair in the gastrointestinal tract [miscellaneous]. Crit Care Med 2003;31:S532–7.
14. Nusrat A, Delp C, Madara JL. Intestinal epithelial restitution. Characterization of a cell culture model and mapping of cytoskeletal elements in migrating cells. J Clin Invest 1992;89:1501–11.
15. Moore R, Carlson S, Madara JL. Rapid barrier restitution in an in vitro model of intestinal epithelial injury. Lab Invest 1989;60:237–44.
16. Dignass AU. Mechanisms and modulation of intestinal epithelial repair. Inflamm Bowel Dis 2001;7:68–77.
17. Grenier A, Chollet-Martin S, Crestani B, et al. Presence of a mobilizable intracellular pool of hepatocyte growth factor in human polymorphonuclear neutrophils. Blood 2002;99:2997–3004.
18. Oka Y, Orth DN. Human plasma epidermal growth factor/beta-urogastrone is associated with blood platelets. J Clin Invest 1983;72:249–59.
19. Karey KP, Marquardt H, Sirbasku DA. Human platelet-derived mitogens. I. Identification of insulinlike growth factors I and II by purification and N alpha amino acid sequence analysis. Blood 1989;74:1084–92.
20. Nakamura T, Nawa K, Ichihara A, et al. Purification and subunit structure of hepatocyte growth factor from rat platelets. FEBS Lett 1987;224:311–6.
21. Playford RJ, Wright NA. Why is epidermal growth factor present in the gut lumen? Gut 1996;38:303–5.

22. Jones MK, Tomikawa M, Mohajer B, et al. Gastrointestinal mucosal regeneration: role of growth factors. Front Biosci 1999;4:D303–9.
23. Abud HE, Watson N, Heath JK. Growth of intestinal epithelium in organ culture is dependent on EGF signalling. Exp Cell Res 2005;303:252–62.
24. Miettinen PJ, Berger JE, Meneses J, et al. Epithelial immaturity and multiorgan failure in mice lacking epidermal growth factor receptor. Nature 1995;376: 337–41.
25. Tepperman BL, Soper BD. Effect of epidermal growth factor, transforming growth factor alpha and nerve growth factor on gastric mucosal integrity and microcirculation in the rat. Regul Pept 1994;50:13–21.
26. Bernal NP, Stehr W, Coyle R, et al. Epidermal growth factor receptor signaling regulates Bax and Bcl-w expression and apoptotic responses during intestinal adaptation in mice. Gastroenterology 2006;130:412–23.
27. Clark JA, Lane RH, Maclennan NK, et al. Epidermal growth factor reduces intestinal apoptosis in an experimental model of necrotizing enterocolitis. Am J Physiol Gastrointest Liver Physiol 2005;288:G755–62.
28. Halpern MD, Dominguez JA, Dvorakova K, et al. Ileal cytokine dysregulation in experimental necrotizing enterocolitis is reduced by epidermal growth factor. J Pediatr Gastroenterol Nutr 2003;36:126–33.
29. Clark JA, Doelle SM, Halpern MD, et al. Intestinal barrier failure during experimental necrotizing enterocolitis: protective effect of EGF treatment. Am J Physiol Gastrointest Liver Physiol 2006;291:G938–49.
30. Clark JA, Gan H, Samocha AJ, et al. Enterocyte-specific epidermal growth factor prevents barrier dysfunction and improves mortality in murine peritonitis. Am J Physiol Gastrointest Liver Physiol 2009;297:G471–9.
31. Clark JA, Clark AT, Hotchkiss RS, et al. Epidermal growth factor treatment decreases mortality and is associated with improved gut integrity in sepsis. Shock 2008;30:36–42.
32. Berlanga J, Prats P, Remirez D, et al. Prophylactic use of epidermal growth factor reduces ischemia/reperfusion intestinal damage. Am J Pathol 2002;161: 373–9.
33. Ishikawa T, Tarnawski A, Sarfeh IJ, et al. Epidermal growth factor protects gastric mucosa against ischemia-reperfusion injury. J Clin Gastroenterol 1993; 17(Suppl 1):S104–10.
34. Berlanga J, Lodos J, Lopez-Saura P. Attenuation of internal organ damages by exogenously administered epidermal growth factor (EGF) in burned rodents. Burns 2002;28:435–42.
35. Dvorak B, Halpern MD, Holubec H, et al. Epidermal growth factor reduces the development of necrotizing enterocolitis in a neonatal rat model. Am J Physiol Gastrointest Liver Physiol 2002;282:G156–64.
36. Erwin CR, Helmrath MA, Shin CE, et al. Intestinal overexpression of EGF in transgenic mice enhances adaptation after small bowel resection. Am J Physiol 1999; 277:G533–40.
37. Chaet MS, Arya G, Ziegler MM, et al. Epidermal growth factor enhances intestinal adaptation after massive small bowel resection. J Pediatr Surg 1994;29: 1035–8.
38. Helmrath MA, Erwin CR, Warner BW. A defective EGF-receptor in waved-2 mice attenuates intestinal adaptation. J Surg Res 1997;69:76–80.
39. Tarnawski A, Stachura J, Durbin T, et al. Increased expression of epidermal growth factor receptor during gastric ulcer healing in rats. Gastroenterology 1992;102:695–8.

40. Itoh M, Matsuo Y. Gastric ulcer treatment with intravenous human epidermal growth factor: a double-blind controlled clinical study. J Gastroenterol Hepatol 1994;9(Suppl 1):S78–83.
41. Clinical trials. Other. 10-19-0009. 10-13-0009. Ref Type: Electronic Citation. Available at: http://clinicaltrials.gov/ct2/results?term=epidermal+growth+factor. Accessed October 13, 2009.
42. Sinha A, Nightingale J, West KP, et al. Epidermal growth factor enemas with oral mesalamine for mild-to-moderate left-sided ulcerative colitis or proctitis. N Engl J Med 2003;349:350–7.
43. Sullivan PB, Lewindon PJ, Cheng C, et al. Intestinal mucosa remodeling by recombinant human epidermal growth factor(1-48) in neonates with severe necrotizing enterocolitis. J Pediatr Surg 2007;42:462–9.
44. Teng CT, Hinds CJ. Treatment with GH and IGF-1 in critical illness. Crit Care Clin 2006;22:29–40, vi.
45. Lang CH, Frost RA. Role of growth hormone, insulin-like growth factor-I, and insulin-like growth factor binding proteins in the catabolic response to injury and infection [miscellaneous article]. Curr Opin Clin Nutr Metab Care 2002;5:271–9.
46. Lal SO, Wolf SE, Herndon DN. Growth hormone, burns and tissue healing. Growth Horm IGF Res 2000;10(Suppl B):S39–43.
47. Briard N, Dadoun F, Pommier G, et al. IGF-I/IGFBPs system response to endotoxin challenge in sheep. J Endocrinol 2000;164:361–9.
48. Dahn MS, Lange MP. Systemic and splanchnic metabolic response to exogenous human growth hormone. Surgery 1998;123:528–38.
49. ehaye-Zervas MC, Mertani H, Martini JF, et al. Expression of the growth hormone receptor gene in human digestive tissue. J Clin Endocrinol Metab 1994;78: 1473–80.
50. Ulshen MH, Dowling RH, Fuller CR, et al. Enhanced growth of small bowel in transgenic mice overexpressing bovine growth hormone. Gastroenterology 1993;104:973–80.
51. Williams KL, Fuller CR, Dieleman LA, et al. Enhanced survival and mucosal repair after dextran sodium sulfate-induced colitis in transgenic mice that overexpress growth hormone. Gastroenterology 2001;120:925–37.
52. Gu Y, Wu ZH, Xie JX, et al. Effects of growth hormone (rhGH) and glutamine supplemented parenteral nutrition on intestinal adaptation in short bowel rats. Clin Nutr 2001;20:159–66.
53. Waitzberg DL, Cukier C, Mucerino DR, et al. Small bowel adaptation with growth hormone and glutamine after massive resection of rat's small bowel. Nutr Hosp 1999;14:81–90.
54. Peterson CA, Gillingham MB, Mohapatra NK, et al. Enterotrophic effect of insulin-like growth factor-I but not growth hormone and localized expression of insulin-like growth factor-I, insulin-like growth factor binding protein-3 and -5 mRNAs in jejunum of parenterally fed rats. JPEN J Parenter Enteral Nutr 2000;24:288–95.
55. Peterson CA, Carey HV, Hinton PL, et al. GH elevates serum IGF-I levels but does not alter mucosal atrophy in parenterally fed rats. Am J Physiol 1997; 272:G1100–8.
56. Jeschke MG, Herndon DN, Finnerty CC, et al. The effect of growth hormone on gut mucosal homeostasis and cellular mediators after severe trauma. J Surg Res 2005;127:183–9.
57. Frost RA, Lang CH. Growth factors in critical illness: regulation and therapeutic aspects [miscellaneous article]. Curr Opin Clin Nutr Metab Care 1998;1: 195–204.

58. Baker J, Liu JP, Robertson EJ, et al. Role of insulin-like growth factors in embryonic and postnatal growth. Cell 1993;75:73–82.

59. Entingh-Pearsall A, Kahn CR. Differential roles of the insulin and insulin-like growth factor-I (IGF-I) receptors in response to insulin and IGF-I. J Biol Chem 2004;279:38016–24.

60. Ohneda K, Ulshen MH, Fuller CR, et al. Enhanced growth of small bowel in transgenic mice expressing human insulin-like growth factor I. Gastroenterology 1997;112:444–54.

61. Zhang W, Frankel WL, Adamson WT, et al. Insulin-like growth factor-I improves mucosal structure and function in transplanted rat small intestine. Transplantation 1995;59:755–61.

62. Huang KF, Chung DH, Herndon DN. Insulinlike growth factor 1 (IGF-1) reduces gut atrophy and bacterial translocation after severe burn injury. Arch Surg 1993; 128:47–53.

63. Fukushima R, Saito H, Inoue T, et al. Prophylactic treatment with growth hormone and insulin-like growth factor I improve systemic bacterial clearance and survival in a murine model of burn-induced gut-derived sepsis. Burns 1999;25:425–30.

64. Ozen S, Akisu M, Baka M, et al. Insulin-like growth factor attenuates apoptosis and mucosal damage in hypoxia/reoxygenation-induced intestinal injury. Biol Neonate 2005;87:91–6.

65. Baregamian N, Song J, Jeschke MG, et al. IGF-1 protects intestinal epithelial cells from oxidative stress-induced apoptosis. J Surg Res 2006;136:31–7.

66. Takala J, Ruokonen E, Webster NR, et al. Increased mortality associated with growth hormone treatment in critically ill adults. N Engl J Med 1999;341:785–92.

67. Taylor BE, Buchman TG. Is there a role for growth hormone therapy in refractory critical illness? Curr Opin Crit Care 2008;14:438–44.

68. Branski LK, Herndon DN, Barrow RE, et al. Randomized controlled trial to determine the efficacy of long-term growth hormone treatment in severely burned children. Ann Surg 2009. [Epub ahead of print]. PMID: 19734776.

69. Jabri N, Schalch DS, Schwartz SL, et al. Adverse effects of recombinant human insulin-like growth factor I in obese insulin-resistant type II diabetic patients. Diabetes 1994;43:369–74.

70. Bondy CA, Underwood LE, Clemmons DR, et al. Clinical uses of insulin-like growth factor I. Ann Intern Med 1994;120:593–601.

71. DebRoy MA, Wolf SE, Zhang XJ, et al. Anabolic effects of insulin-like growth factor in combination with insulin-like growth factor binding protein-3 in severely burned adults. J Trauma 1999;47:904–10.

72. Herndon DN, Ramzy PI, DebRoy MA, et al. Muscle protein catabolism after severe burn: effects of IGF-1/IGFBP-3 treatment. Ann Surg 1999;229: 713–20.

73. Jeschke MG, Barrow RE, Suzuki F, et al. IGF-I/IGFBP-3 equilibrates ratios of pro- to anti-inflammatory cytokines, which are predictors for organ function in severely burned pediatric patients. Mol Med 2002;8:238–46.

74. Jeschke MG, Barrow RE, Herndon DN. Insulinlike growth factor I plus insulinlike growth factor binding protein 3 attenuates the proinflammatory acute phase response in severely burned children. Ann Surg 2000;231:246–52.

75. Jeschke MG, Bolder U, Chung DH, et al. Gut mucosal homeostasis and cellular mediators after severe thermal trauma and the effect of insulin-like growth factor-I in combination with insulin-like growth factor binding protein-3. Endocrinology 2007;148:354–62.

76. Finch PW, Rubin JS, Miki T, et al. Human KGF is FGF-related with properties of a paracrine effector of epithelial cell growth. Science 1989;245:752–5.
77. Brauchle M, Madlener M, Wagner AD, et al. Keratinocyte growth factor is highly overexpressed in inflammatory bowel disease. Am J Pathol 1996;149:521–9.
78. Housley RM, Morris CF, Boyle W, et al. Keratinocyte growth factor induces proliferation of hepatocytes and epithelial cells throughout the rat gastrointestinal tract. J Clin Invest 1994;94:1764–77.
79. Zeeh JM, Procaccino F, Hoffmann P, et al. Keratinocyte growth factor ameliorates mucosal injury in an experimental model of colitis in rats. Gastroenterology 1996;110:1077–83.
80. Chen Y, Chou K, Fuchs E, et al. Protection of the intestinal mucosa by intraepithelial gamma delta T cells. Proc Natl Acad Sci U S A 2002;99:14338–43.
81. Wildhaber BE, Yang H, Teitelbaum DH. Keratinocyte growth factor decreases total parenteral nutrition-induced apoptosis in mouse intestinal epithelium via Bcl-2. J Pediatr Surg 2003;38:92–6.
82. Finch PW, Rubin JS. Keratinocyte growth factor/fibroblast growth factor 7, a homeostatic factor with therapeutic potential for epithelial protection and repair. Adv Cancer Res 2004;91:69–136.
83. Khan WB, Shui C, Ning S, et al. Enhancement of murine intestinal stem cell survival after irradiation by keratinocyte growth factor. Radiat Res 1997;148: 248–53.
84. Farrell CL, Bready JV, Rex KL, et al. Keratinocyte growth factor protects mice from chemotherapy and radiation-induced gastrointestinal injury and mortality. Cancer Res 1998;58:933–9.
85. Sandborn WJ, Sands BE, Wolf DC, et al. Repifermin (keratinocyte growth factor-2) for the treatment of active ulcerative colitis: a randomized, double-blind, placebo-controlled, dose-escalation trial. Aliment Pharmacol Ther 2003;17: 1355–64.
86. Kanayama M, Takahara T, Yata Y, et al. Hepatocyte growth factor promotes colonic epithelial regeneration via Akt signaling. Am J Physiol Gastrointest Liver Physiol 2007;293:G230–9.
87. Ido A, Numata M, Kodama M, et al. Mucosal repair and growth factors: recombinant human hepatocyte growth factor as an innovative therapy for inflammatory bowel disease. J Gastroenterol 2005;40:925–31.
88. Nishimura S, Takahashi M, Ota S, et al. Hepatocyte growth factor accelerates restitution of intestinal epithelial cells. J Gastroenterol 1998;33:172–8.
89. Schwartz MZ, Kato Y, Yu D, et al. Growth-factor enhancement of compromised gut function following massive small-bowel resection. Pediatr Surg Int 2000;16: 174–5.
90. Jeschke MG, Bolder U, Finnerty CC, et al. The effect of hepatocyte growth factor on gut mucosal apoptosis and proliferation, and cellular mediators after severe trauma. Surgery 2005;138:482–9.
91. Kuenzler KA, Pearson PY, Schwartz MZ. Hepatocyte growth factor pretreatment reduces apoptosis and mucosal damage after intestinal ischemia-reperfusion. J Pediatr Surg 2002;37:1093–7.
92. Tahara Y, Ido A, Yamamoto S, et al. Hepatocyte growth factor facilitates colonic mucosal repair in experimental ulcerative colitis in rats. J Pharmacol Exp Ther 2003;307:146–51.
93. Numata M, Ido A, Moriuchi A, et al. Hepatocyte growth factor facilitates the repair of large colonic ulcers in 2,4,6-trinitrobenzene sulfonic acid-induced colitis in rats. Inflamm Bowel Dis 2005;11:551–8.

94. Ohda Y, Hori K, Tomita T, et al. Effects of hepatocyte growth factor on rat inflammatory bowel disease models. Dig Dis Sci 2005;50:914–21.
95. Mukoyama T, Kanbe T, Murai R, et al. Therapeutic effect of adenoviral-mediated hepatocyte growth factor gene administration on TNBS-induced colitis in mice. Biochem Biophys Res Commun 2005;329:1217–24.
96. Kanbe T, Murai R, Mukoyama T, et al. Naked gene therapy of hepatocyte growth factor for dextran sulfate sodium-induced colitis in mice. Biochem Biophys Res Commun 2006;345:1517–25.
97. Hanawa T, Suzuki K, Kawauchi Y, et al. Attenuation of mouse acute colitis by naked hepatocyte growth factor gene transfer into the liver. J Gene Med 2006;8:623–35.
98. Oh K, Iimuro Y, Takeuchi M, et al. Ameliorating effect of hepatocyte growth factor on inflammatory bowel disease in a murine model. Am J Physiol Gastrointest Liver Physiol 2005;288:G729–35.
99. Sakata H, Takayama H, Sharp R, et al. Hepatocyte growth factor/scatter factor overexpression induces growth, abnormal development, and tumor formation in transgenic mouse livers. Cell Growth Differ 1996;7:1513–23.
100. Higashiyama S, Abraham JA, Miller J, et al. A heparin-binding growth factor secreted by macrophage-like cells that is related to EGF. Science 1991;251:936–9.
101. vis-Fleischer KM, Besner GE. Structure and function of heparin-binding EGF-like growth factor (HB-EGF). Front Biosci 1998;3:d288–99.
102. Cribbs RK, Harding PA, Luquette MH, et al. Endogenous production of heparin-binding EGF-like growth factor during murine partial-thickness burn wound healing. J Burn Care Rehabil 2002;23:116–25.
103. Michalsky MP, Kuhn A, Mehta V, et al. Heparin-binding EGF-like growth factor decreases apoptosis in intestinal epithelial cells in vitro. J Pediatr Surg 2001;36:1130–5.
104. Pillai SB, Turman MA, Besner GE. Heparin-binding EGF-like growth factor is cytoprotective for intestinal epithelial cells exposed to hypoxia. J Pediatr Surg 1998;33:973–8.
105. Kuhn MA, Xia G, Mehta VB, et al. Heparin-binding EGF-like growth factor (HB-EGF) decreases oxygen free radical production in vitro and in vivo. Antioxid Redox Signal 2002;4:639–46.
106. Xia G, Martin AE, Michalsky MP, et al. Heparin-binding EGF-like growth factor preserves crypt cell proliferation and decreases bacterial translocation after intestinal ischemia/reperfusion injury. J Pediatr Surg 2002;37:1081–7.
107. Feng J, Besner GE. Heparin-binding epidermal growth factor-like growth factor promotes enterocyte migration and proliferation in neonatal rats with necrotizing enterocolitis. J Pediatr Surg 2007;42:214–20.
108. El-Assal ON, Radulescu A, Besner GE. Heparin-binding EGF-like growth factor preserves mesenteric microcirculatory blood flow and protects against intestinal injury in rats subjected to hemorrhagic shock and resuscitation. Surgery 2007;142:234–42.
109. Brubaker PL, Drucker DJ. Minireview: glucagon-like peptides regulate cell proliferation and apoptosis in the pancreas, gut, and central nervous system. Endocrinology 2004;145:2653–9.
110. Scott RB, Kirk D, MacNaughton WK, et al. GLP-2 augments the adaptive response to massive intestinal resection in rat. Am J Physiol 1998;275:G911–21.
111. Sigalet DL, Martin GR. Hormonal therapy for short bowel syndrome. J Pediatr Surg 2000;35:360–3.

112. Alavi K, Schwartz MZ, Palazzo JP, et al. Treatment of inflammatory bowel disease in a rodent model with the intestinal growth factor glucagon-like peptide-2. J Pediatr Surg 2000;35:847–51.

113. L'Heureux MC, Brubaker PL. Glucagon-like peptide-2 and common therapeutics in a murine model of ulcerative colitis. J Pharmacol Exp Ther 2003;306: 347–54.

114. Boushey RP, Yusta B, Drucker DJ. Glucagon-like peptide 2 decreases mortality and reduces the severity of indomethacin-induced murine enteritis. Am J Physiol 1999;277:E937–47.

115. Cameron HL, Yang PC, Perdue MH. Glucagon-like peptide-2-enhanced barrier function reduces pathophysiology in a model of food allergy. Am J Physiol Gastrointest Liver Physiol 2003;284:G905–12.

116. Benjamin MA, McKay DM, Yang PC, et al. Glucagon-like peptide-2 enhances intestinal epithelial barrier function of both transcellular and paracellular pathways in the mouse. Gut 2000;47:112–9.

117. Kouris GJ, Liu Q, Rossi H, et al. The effect of glucagon-like peptide 2 on intestinal permeability and bacterial translocation in acute necrotizing pancreatitis. Am J Surg 2001;181:571–5.

118. Chance WT, Sheriff S, McCarter F, et al. Glucagon-like peptide-2 stimulates gut mucosal growth and immune response in burned rats. J Burn Care Rehabil 2001;22:136–43.

119. Rajeevprasad R, Alavi K, Schwartz MZ. Glucagonlike peptide-2 analogue enhances intestinal mucosal mass and absorptive function after ischemia-reperfusion injury. J Pediatr Surg 2000;35:1537–9.

120. Drucker DJ, Yusta B, Boushey RP, et al. Human [Gly2]GLP-2 reduces the severity of colonic injury in a murine model of experimental colitis. Am J Physiol 1999;276:G79–91.

121. Burrin DG, Stoll B, Jiang R, et al. GLP-2 stimulates intestinal growth in premature TPN-fed pigs by suppressing proteolysis and apoptosis. Am J Physiol Gastrointest Liver Physiol 2000;279:G1249–56.

122. Burrin DG, Stoll B, Guan X, et al. GLP-2 rapidly activates divergent intracellular signaling pathways involved in intestinal cell survival and proliferation in neonatal piglets. Am J Physiol Endocrinol Metab 2007;292:E281–91.

123. Jeppesen PB, Hartmann B, Thulesen J, et al. Glucagon-like peptide 2 improves nutrient absorption and nutritional status in short-bowel patients with no colon. Gastroenterology 2001;120:806–15.

124. Thim L. Trefoil peptides: a new family of gastrointestinal molecules. Digestion 1994;55:353–60.

125. Babyatsky MW, deBeaumont M, Thim L, et al. Oral trefoil peptides protect against ethanol- and indomethacin-induced gastric injury in rats. Gastroenterology 1996;110:489–97.

126. Cook GA, Thim L, Yeomans ND, et al. Oral human spasmolytic polypeptide protects against aspirin-induced gastric injury in rats. J Gastroenterol Hepatol 1998;13:363–70.

127. Tran CP, Cook GA, Yeomans ND, et al. Trefoil peptide TFF2 (spasmolytic polypeptide) potently accelerates healing and reduces inflammation in a rat model of colitis. Gut 1999;44:636–42.

128. Taupin DR, Kinoshita K, Podolsky DK. Intestinal trefoil factor confers colonic epithelial resistance to apoptosis. Proc Natl Acad Sci U S A 2000;97:799–804.

129. Sands BE, Podolsky DK. The trefoil peptide family. Annu Rev Physiol 1996;58: 253–73.

130. Mashimo H, Wu DC, Podolsky DK, et al. Impaired defense of intestinal mucosa in mice lacking intestinal trefoil factor. Science 1996;274:262–5.
131. Shi L, Zhang BH, Yu HG, et al. Intestinal trefoil factor in treatment of neonatal necrotizing enterocolitis in the rat model. J Perinat Med 2007;35:443–6.
132. Vandenbroucke K, Hans W, Van HJ, et al. Active delivery of trefoil factors by genetically modified *Lactococcus lactis* prevents and heals acute colitis in mice. Gastroenterology 2004;127:502–13.
133. Beck PL, Wong JF, Li Y, et al. Chemotherapy- and radiotherapy-induced intestinal damage is regulated by intestinal trefoil factor. Gastroenterology 2004;126: 796–808.
134. Sun YM, Wu WM, Zhang YM, et al. Intestinal trefoil factor produced in *Escherichia coli* promotes the healing of rat burn-induced acute gastric mucosal lesions [article]. J Trauma 2008;65:163–9.
135. Yong S, Wu W, Zhang Y, et al. Stability analysis of recombinant human TFF2 and its therapeutic effect on burn-induced gastric injury in mice. Burns 2009;35: 869–74.
136. Cibrian D, Ajamieh H, Berlanga J, et al. Use of growth-hormone-releasing peptide-6 (GHRP-6) for the prevention of multiple organ failure. Clin Sci (Lond) 2006;110:563–73.
137. Jacobs DO, Evans DA, Mealy K, et al. Combined effects of glutamine and epidermal growth factor on the rat intestine. Surgery 1988;104:358–64.
138. Ko TC, Beauchamp RD, Townsend CM Jr, et al. Glutamine is essential for epidermal growth factor-stimulated intestinal cell proliferation. Surgery 1993; 114:147–53.
139. Zhang W, Bain A, Rombeau JL. Insulin-like growth factor-I (IGF-I) and glutamine improve structure and function in the small bowel allograft. J Surg Res 1995;59: 6–12.
140. Byrne TA, Morrissey TB, Nattakom TV, et al. Growth hormone, glutamine, and a modified diet enhance nutrient absorption in patients with severe short bowel syndrome. JPEN J Parenter Enteral Nutr 1995;19:296–302.

Mitochondrial Dysfunction and Resuscitation in Sepsis

Albert J. Ruggieri, BS[a,c], Richard J. Levy, MD[b,c], Clifford S. Deutschman, MS, MD, FCCM[a,c,*]

KEYWORDS

- Sepsis • Mitochondria • Mitochondrial dysfunction
- Cytopathic hypoxia • Electron transport • Cytochrome c • ATP

Sepsis is among the most common causes of death in patients in the intensive care unit in North America and Europe. In the United States it accounts for upwards of 250,000 deaths each year.[1] Nonetheless, the importance of sepsis as a public health problem is underappreciated; this partly stems from changing definitions. The dictionary definition invokes the presence of dividing microorganisms in the blood, but this has proven to be too narrow. The first systematic approach to the classification of sepsis, the 1992 Society of Critical Care Medicine (SCCM)/American College of Chest Physicians Consensus Conference, clarified some of the diagnostic criteria and also first introduced the concept of the systemic inflammatory response syndrome.[2] This entity was defined based on temperature, heart rate, respiratory rate, and white blood cell counts. Although useful in defining entry criteria for clinical studies, this approach has proven to be too general and nonspecific. Therefore, the 2001 revision jointly sponsored by the SCCM and the European Society of Intensive Care Medicine is based on the presence of general variables, inflammatory variables, hemodynamics, organ dysfunction, and tissue perfusion.

The concept that sepsis necessarily involves infection has been eliminated, which is important for two reasons. First, no organism is ever identified in upwards of 50% of patients who die with a diagnosis of sepsis. Second, systemic infection and similar inflammatory states give rise to a more recently appreciated entity, the multiple organ

[a] Department of Anesthesiology and Critical Care, University of Pennsylvania School of Medicine, Philadelphia, PA 19104-4283, USA
[b] Division of Anesthesiology and Pain Medicine, Children's National Medical Center, Washington, DC 20010, USA
[c] The Stavropoulos Sepsis Research Program, University of Pennsylvania School of Medicine, Philadelphia, PA 19104-4283, USA
* Corresponding author. Dulles 781A/HUP, 3400 Spruce Street, Philadelphia, PA 19104-4283.
E-mail address: deutschcl@uphs.upenn.edu

Crit Care Clin 26 (2010) 567–575
doi:10.1016/j.ccc.2010.04.007   criticalcare.theclinics.com
0749-0704/10/$ – see front matter © 2010 Elsevier Inc. All rights reserved.

dysfunction syndrome (MODS).[3] This clinically defined common final pathway may develop in patients with severe infection but also after severe trauma, aortic aneurysm rupture, amniotic fluid embolism, and a host of other conditions. The development of MODS suggests that the pathogenesis of sepsis cannot be attributed solely to invading organisms but rather must reflect the host response to some severe insult. The search for a primary defect and the mechanism through which it impairs function in a broad array of cells and organs has been the focus of intense investigation for several decades.

MITOCHONDRIAL FUNCTION AND ENERGY PRODUCTION

Investigations into the pathobiology of sepsis have most recently focused on cellular and subcellular processes that are common to most cells and organs. One possibility would be a defect in the production of energy, which translates to an abnormality in the production of adenosine triphosphate (ATP) and therefore in the function of mitochondria.

Mitochondria are cellular organelles characterized by a unique double-membrane structure that maintain intracellular homeostasis through several key functions. Most important of these is the production of energy that can then be consumed elsewhere in the cell. In this process, ATP is produced from adenosine diphosphate (ADP) and consumed. A description of normal mitochondrial function is required before studies examining mitochondrial failure can be entertained as a cause of septic pathophysiology and the development of MODS.

The initiation of mitochondrial energy production in fact does not occur in mitochondria but most often occurs in the cytoplasm. This process, glycolysis (**Fig. 1**), is a series of reactions through which glucose (derived most often from food but also synthesized by organs such as the liver and the kidney) is phosphorylated twice, cleaved, and ultimately rearranged to form two pyruvate molecules.

Pyruvate can be used in several ways. One common pathway involves the continuation of cytoplasmic glycolysis, with pyruvate being converted to lactate by the enzyme lactate dehydrogenase, producing two ATP molecules per molecule of pyruvate. Most often, and in the presence of oxygen, however, pyruvate enters mitochondria through pyruvate dehydrogenase, is converted to acetate, linked to coenzyme A to form acetyl coenzyme A (acetyl-CoA), and combined with oxaloacetate to form citrate. The process through which citrate contributes to the process, also called the citric acid cycle, tricarboxylic acid cycle, or Krebs cycle (after Hans Krebs, the biochemist who, along with Albert Szent-Gyorgyi, first described the process), involves enzymes located within the mitochondrial matrix (**Fig. 2**). During these enzymatic reactions, reducing equivalents are created and stored in the form of nicotinamide adenine dinucleotide dihydride (NADH-H$^+$), flavin adenine dinucleotide hydride (FADH2+), or coenzyme Q (CoQ). The net energy product from the Krebs cycle is minor. However, the electron carriers (FADH$_2$, NADH-H$^+$, and CoQ) provide substrate for the electron transport chain.

The electron transport chain (**Fig. 3**) transfers energy from carriers to form ATP. This is accomplished by passing the energy, in the form of electrons, through four protein complexes on the inner mitochondrial membrane. Coupled with electron transport, protons (H$^+$) are pumped into the intramembrane space by complexes I, III, and IV. The result is an electrochemical potential gradient, $\Delta\Psi_m$, of 180 mV. The energy from $\Delta\Psi_m$ is used by the fifth complex, ATP synthase, to convert ADP to high-energy ATP. The mobile electron-carrying molecules within the chain are ubiquinone and cytochrome c. In complex IV, cytochrome c oxidase, electrons from cytochrome c

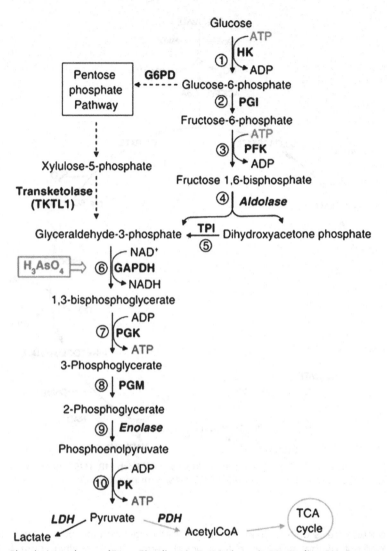

Fig. 1. Glycolytic pathway. (*From* Zivadinovic D, Marjanovic M, Andjus RK. Some components of hibernation rhythms. Ann N Y Acad Sci 2005;1048:60–8; with permission.)

are transferred to molecular oxygen. The O_2^{-2} combines with two H^+ ions to form water.

It is well understood that active release of cytochrome c into the cytoplasm can initiate apoptosis, or programmed cell death. However, data suggest that this does not occur in sepsis within most organs. In aerobic environments, the amount of ATP that can be produced may be limited only by the availability of pyruvate. To limit the proton gradient from becoming excessive, a controlled leak back into the mitochondrial matrix is mediated by carriers called *uncoupling proteins*.

The most profound disruption of the proton-motive force and normal mitochondrial function occurs when the mitochondrial membrane becomes excessively permeable.

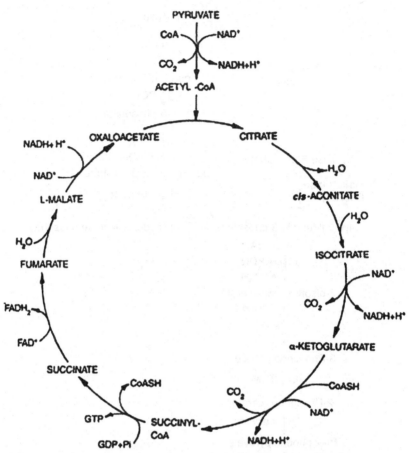

Fig. 2. Citric acid cycle. (*From* Blackstone E, Morrison M, Roth MB. H2S induces a suspended animation-like state in mice. Science 2005;308:518; with permission.)

This occurrence is characteristic of several pathologic conditions and leads to the development of the so-called mitochondrial permeability transition pore (MPTP), a large, nonspecific channel in the internal mitochondrial membrane. MPTP opening (called *mitochondrial permeability transition*) allows water and molecules of up to 1.5 kDa to cross the usually impermeable internal membrane. The resulting depolarization uncouples oxidative phosphorylation, depletes ATP, promotes mitochondrial swelling, and may initiate apoptosis.

Under normal conditions, mitochondria are destroyed and replaced on a regular basis. Destruction occurs by autophagy. Regeneration of mitochondria, called *biogenesis,* is a tightly regulated process that involves expression of a set of proteins, transfer RNAs, and ribosomal RNAs that are encoded by DNA contained within the mitochondria (mtDNA). mtRNA expression, in turn, is controlled by a complex series of reactions that may involve the expression of upwards of 1000 nuclear-encoded proteins. Failed biogenesis is another source of profound disruption of mitochondrial function that is seen in pathologic states, including sepsis.

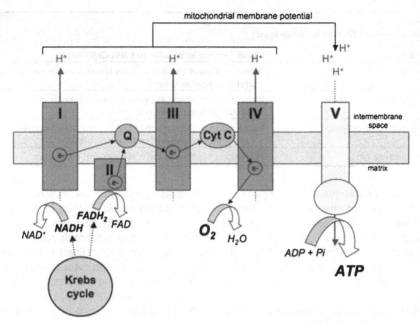

Fig. 3. The electron transport chain. (*From* Burwell LS, Nadtochiy SM, Brookes PS. Cardioprotection by metabolic shut-down and gradual wake-up. J Mol Cell Cardiol 2009;46:804–10; with permission.)

MITOCHONDRIAL DYSFUNCTION IN SEPSIS
Oxygen Use and ATP Dynamics

Mitochondrial impairment during critical illness has been recognized for some time. Hypoxia-induced mitochondrial dysfunction was first identified by Barcroft and colleagues[4] in 1945. This investigation identified three causes of hypoxia that led to mitochondrial dysfunction: decreased arterial oxygen tension (hypoxic hypoxia), decreased systemic hemoglobin concentration (anemic hypoxia), and microvascular dysfunction leading to hypoperfusion (stagnant hypoxia). However, the effects of sepsis on cellular ATP levels are unclear. Work by Hotchkiss and Karl[5] in skeletal muscle suggests that sepsis depletes cellular ATP content, not from a lack of oxygen but rather because high-energy phosphate levels may be reduced. In contrast, studies on muscle and liver by Brealey and colleagues[6] did not show ATP depletion.[7] Most importantly, recent investigations clearly show that sepsis impairs ATP production.[8] Therefore, the maintenance of normal levels must reflect decreased use.

Microvascular Dysfunction Versus Cytopathic Hypoxia

Initial research regarding septic pathophysiology led clinicians to propose that the key abnormality was microvascular dysfunction. This entity, involving a heterogeneous alteration in perfusion, was first described by Weil and Shubin,[9] in 1971. The perfusion mismatch would result in failed peripheral oxygen use.[10] Sidestream dark-field imaging has revealed an impaired microcirculation in septic patients.[10] Using this approach, Ince and colleagues[10] found that capillary perfusion in sepsis may take any combination of five forms (**Table 1**). The net effect is a failure of oxygen delivery in sepsis.

Table 1 Microvascular flow patterns in sepsis	
Stagnant	**Blood Moving in Venules but Not Capillaries**
Empty/continuous	Blood moving in venules with no blood in some capillaries and free flow in others
Stagnant/continuous	Blood moving in venules with impaired flow in some capillaries and free flow in others
Stagnant/hyperdynamic	Hyperdynamic flow in venules, stagnant flow in some capillaries and hyperdynamically in others
Hyperdynamic	Hyperdynamic flow in both venules and capillaries.

Fink and colleagues[7,11,12] proposed that microvascular dysfunction may not be the abnormality that effects mitochondrial respiration during sepsis. Rather, flow may be normal or even excessive, but an intrinsic derangement affecting cellular energy metabolism may preclude oxygen use. This defect is called *cytopathic hypoxia* and its existence is supported by tissue oxygen measurements and direct examination of cellular and mitochondrial respiration. Mechanisms that explain cytopathic hypoxia during sepsis include impaired pyruvate delivery, inhibition of the enzymes involved in Krebs cycle or the electron transport chain, activation of poly(ADP-ribosyl) polymerase (PARP), and failed maintenance of the transmitochondrial membrane proton gradient with uncoupling of ATP synthase.[7]

Pyruvate Dehydrogenase Dysfunction

Pyruvate dehydrogenase (PDH) E1 is a catalytic component of the multimeric pyruvate dehydrogenase complex (PDC) that is responsible for synthesizing acetyl-CoA from pyruvate. PDH activity is stimulated by insulin, phosphoenolpyruvic acid and AMP and is inhibited by ATP, nicotinamide adenine dinucleotide, and acetyl-CoA. Inactivation of the PDC will inevitably impair ATP production.[13]

PDC dysfunction in sepsis was at one time the subject of intense investigation,[14] which showed increased lactate production despite normal to increased skeletal muscle blood flow. Similarly, in the liver of rats made septic by cecal ligation and puncture (CLP), Kantrow and colleagues[15] found decreased oxygen consumption and attributed this to failed generation of substrate (glutamate, malate, succinate) for the Krebs cycle/electron transport chain.[16] Interest in PDH and the elements of the Krebs cycle has waned as focus has shifted to components of the electron transport chain. However, the abnormalities in electron transport may be adaptive, which makes it increasingly important to identify other defects.

Altered Oxidative Phosphorylation

Impaired ATP production could result from dysfunction in any of the four complexes of the electron transport chain. These complexes develop a proton gradient that creates the energy potential used by ATP synthase to convert ADP into ATP.[11,12,17] The cycle of production and consumption continues as long as glucose is fed into the system and respiration is not inhibited.

Cytochrome c oxidase, complex IV of the electron transport chain, consists of 13 different subunits, three of which constitute the active site where O^{-2} combines with 2 H^+ molecules to form water. This action also helps generate the electrical intermembrane potential for ATP generation. The active site is characterized by a copper-containing center and two heme centers (heme a, a3) where molecular oxygen is bound. Because of its role as the final electron acceptor and the complex that uses oxygen, complex IV is believed by many to be of prime importance, and perhaps even rate-limited. Studies in murine models of sepsis have shown noncompetitive inhibition of cytochrome c use. At late time points, loss of heme content and failure of subunit I expression occur.[18] The active subunits are encoded by mtDNA. A decrease in the abundance of these key subunits likely indicates failed biogenesis and irreversible mitochondrial dysfunction.

Experimentally, the activity of complex II is difficult to separate from that of complex III. Therefore, most studies report on joint activity. Several investigations show sepsis-associated dysfunction of complex II/III. Brealey and colleagues[6] studied electron transport activity using a rodent model of sepsis. They were unable to identify a defect in complex II/III activity in either liver or skeletal muscle over 72 hours. However, activity of hepatic complex I and IV fell over time. At the late time point in septic animals, all complex protein activity was noted to be much lower than sham-operated mice in both hepatic and muscle tissue.

Fredriksson and colleagues[19] studied mitochondrial metabolic dysfunction in septic patients in the intensive care unit and compared this with healthy patients undergoing elective surgery. In septic patients experiencing MODS they observed a twofold decrease in all mitochondrial complex activity in intercostal muscle and leg muscle.

Inhibition of either complex I or IV can increase the production of reactive oxygen (ROS) and nitric oxide (NO).[20–24] Production of these free radicals increases with aging and in individuals with immune dysfunction.[25] Both have been implicated in the pathogenesis of sepsis when excess production may overwhelm endogenous protective mechanisms[24] and impair mitochondrial bioenergetic production.[22,23] ROS and NO in excess also may induce mitochondrially mediated apoptosis.

RESUSCITATION

Complex IV is inhibited in septic mice. Piel and colleagues,[26] administered exogenous cytochrome c (cyt c) and examined the effect on mitochondrial dysfunction and myocardial contractility. These studies showed that cyt c given 24 hours after the induction of sepsis through CLP abrogated the inhibition of complex IV and improved cardiac contractility. Furthermore, 50% of cyt c–injected mice survived to 96 hours in contrast to only 15% in saline-injected mice.[27] Despite the demonstrated role of cyt c in apoptosis, no increase in programmed cell death was noted.

In addition to exogenous cyt c, the authors examined the effects of caffeine on sepsis-induced mitochondrial dysfunction. Verma and colleagues[28] showed that the intraperitoneal injection of 7.5 mg/kg of caffeine (equivalent to the concentration in an average cup of coffee) in mice after CLP increased complex IV kinetic activity to levels equivalent to those seen after sham operation.

SUMMARY: IS EARLY SEPSIS-INDUCED MITOCHONDRIAL INHIBITION ADAPTIVE?

The data discussed show a clear role for mitochondrial dysfunction in the pathogenesis and pathophysiology of sepsis. What is less clear is the teleology underlying this response. Prolonged mitochondrial dysfunction and impaired biogenesis clearly are detrimental. However, early inhibition of mitochondrial function may serve another purpose.

After experimental ischemia-reperfusion injury and clinically after myocardial infarction, the heart enters a state of reduced metabolism and contractility. This response is referred to as *hibernation* and is viewed to be adaptive, allowing demarcation of irreversibly effected muscle and recovery of tissue that is incompletely effected.[29] Use of hydrogen sulfide[30] and S-nitrosothiols,[31–34] which inhibit complex IV and I, respectively, have been shown to induce a similar state and protect against ischemia-reperfusion injury. It is attractive to postulate that sepsis-induced reductions in organ function are similarly protective.[17] This concept, termed *metabolic quiescence* proposes that, in response to some sepsis-induced injury, the production of NO, carbon monoxide (CO), or some other molecular species that binds to the heme moiety in complex IV reversibly inhibits the function of this enzyme. This hypothesis is supported by the sepsis-induced (1) overproduction of NO and CO, (2) decrease in ATP production,[8] (3) lack of irreversible damage after recovery, (4) demonstration of noncompetitive inhibition of complex IV in septic myocardium[18] and liver (Deutschman CS, unpublished data, 2010), and (5) demonstration of increased glycogen deposition, enhanced expression of the GLUT4 receptor, and a switch in myocardial substrate preference from fatty acids to glucose, all characteristic of hibernation after ischemia-reperfusion injury.

The "mitochondrial inhibition as an adaptive response" hypothesis is intriguing but remains unproven. What is clear is that investigation into the role of mitochondria in the pathogenesis and pathophysiology of sepsis represents an exciting avenue of future investigation.

REFERENCES

1. Angus DC, Linde-Zwirble WT, Lidicker J, et al. Epidemiology of severe sepsis in the United States: analysis of incidence, outcome, and associated costs of care. Crit Care Med 2001;29:1303–10.
2. Members of the American College of Chest Physicians/Society of Critical Care Consensus Committee; American College of Chest Physicians/Society of Critical Care Medicine Consensus Conference. Definitions of sepsis and organ failure and guidelines for the use of innovative therapies in sepsis. Crit Care Med 1992;20:864–74.
3. Levy MM, Fink MP, Marshall JC, et al. 2001 SCCM/ESICM/ACCP/ATS/SIS International sepsis definition conference. Crit Care Med 2003;31:1250–6.
4. Barcroft H, Allen WJ, Anderson DP, et al. Circulatory changes during fainting and coma caused by oxygen lack. J Physiol 1946;104:426–34.
5. Hotchkiss RS, Karl IE. Reevaluation of the role of cellular hypoxia and bioenergetic failure in sepsis. JAMA 1992;267:1503–10.
6. Brealey D, Karyampudi S, Jacques TS, et al. Mitochondrial dysfunction in a long-term rodent model of sepsis and organ failure. Am J Phys 2004;286:R491–7.
7. Fink MP. Cytopathic hypoxia: mitochondrial dysfunction as mechanism contributing to organ dysfunction in sepsis. Crit Care Clin 2001;17:219–37.
8. López LC, Escames G, Ortiz F, et al. Melatonin restores the mitochondrial production of ATP in septic mice. Neuro Endocrinol Lett 2006;27:623–30.
9. Weil MH, Shubin H. Proposed reclassification of shock states with special reference to distributive effects. Advance Experiments in Medical Biology 1971;23: 13–23.
10. Elbers PW, Ince C. Bench-to-bedside review: mechanisms of critical illness—classifying microcirculatory flow abnormalities in distributive shock. Crit Care Clin 2006;10:221.
11. Fink MP. Bench-to-bedside review: cytopathic hypoxia. Crit Care Clin 2002;6: 491–9.
12. Fink MP. Cytopathic hypoxia. Is oxygen use impaired in sepsis as a result of acquired intrinsic derangement in cellular respiration? Crit Care Clin 2002;18: 165–75.

13. Vary TC, Siegel JH, Nakatani T, et al. Effect on sepsis on activity of pyruvate dehydrogenase complex in skeletal muscle and liver. Am J Physiol Endocrinol Metab 1986;250:E634–40.
14. Vary TC, Hazen S. Sepsis alters pyruvate dehydrogenase kinase activity in skeletal muscle. Mol Cell Biochem 1999;198:113–8.
15. Kantrow SP, Taylor DE, Carraway MS, et al. Oxidative metabolism in rat hepatocytes and mitochondria during sepsis. Arch Biochem Biophys 1997;345:278–88.
16. Kantrow SP, Tatro LG, Piantidosi CA. Oxidative stress and adenine nucleotide control of mitochondrial permeability transition. Free Radic Biol Med 2000;28:251–60.
17. Levy RJ. Mitochondrial dysfunction, bioenergetic impairment, and metabolic down-regulation in sepsis. Shock 2007;28:24–8.
18. Levy RJ, Vijayasarathy C, Raj NR, et al. Competitive and noncompetitive inhibition of myocardial cytochrome c oxidase in sepsis. Shock 2004;21:110–4.
19. Fredriksson K, Hammarqvist F, Strigard K, et al. Derangements in mitochondrial metabolism in intercostal and leg muscle of critically ill patients with sepsis-induced multiple organ failure. Am J Phys 2006;291:E1044–50.
20. Brealey D, Brand M, Hargreaves L, et al. Association between mitochondrial dysfunction and severity and outcome of septic shock. Lancet 2002;360:219–23.
21. Clementi E, Brown GC, Feelisch M, et al. Persistent inhibition of cell respiration by nitric oxide: crucial role of S-nitrosylation of mitochondrial complex I and protective action of glutathione. Proc Natl Acad Sci U S A 1998;95:7631–6.
22. Bolanos JP, Heales SJ, Peuchen S, et al. Nitric oxide-mediated mitochondrial damage: a potential neuroprotective role for glutathione. Free Radic Biol Med 1996;21:995–1001.
23. Hoffman DL, Brookes PS. Oxygen sensitivity of mitochondrial reactive oxygen species generation depends on metabolic conditions. J Biol Chem 2009;284:16236–45.
24. Taylor DE, Ghio AJ, Piantadosi CA. Reactive oxygen species produced by liver mitochondria of rats in sepsis. Arch Biochem Biophys 1995;316:70–6.
25. Rada B, Leto TL. Oxidative innate immune defenses by Nox/Duox family NADPH oxidases. Contrib Microbiol 2008;15:164–87.
26. Piel DA, Gruber PJ, Weinheimer CJ, et al. Mitochondrial resuscitation with exogenous cytochrome c in the septic heart. Crit Care Med 2007;35:2120–7.
27. Piel DA, Deutschman CS, Levy RJ. Exogenous cytochrome c restores myocardial cytochrome oxidase activity into the late phase of sepsis. Shock 2008;29:612–6.
28. Verma R, Huang Z, Deutschman CS, et al. Caffeine restores myocardial cytochrome oxidase activity and improves cardiac function during sepsis. Crit Care Med 2009;37:1397–402.
29. Zivadinovic D, Marjanovic M, Andjus RK. Some components of hibernation rhythms. Ann N Y Acad Sci 2005;1048:60–8.
30. Blackstone E, Morrison M, Roth MB. H2S induces a suspended animation-like state in mice. Science 2005;308:518.
31. Burwell LS, Nadtochiy SM, Brookes PS. Cardioprotection by metabolic shut-down and gradual wake-up. J Mol Cell Cardiol 2009;46:804–10.
32. Pelicano H, Martin DS, Xu RH, et al. Glycolysis inhibition for anticancer treatment. Oncogene 2006;25:4633–46.
33. Bender DA, Mayes PA. Glycolysis and the oxidation of pyruvate; Harper's illustrated biochemistry. 28th edition. The McGraw-Hill Companies; 2009.
34. Protti A, Singer M. Bench-to-bedside review: potential strategies to protect or reverse mitochondrial dysfunction in sepsis-induced organ failure. Crit Care Forum 2006;10:228.

Index

Note: Page numbers of article titles are in **boldface** type.

A

Acid(s), fatty, omega-3. See *Omega-3 fatty acids.*
Altered oxidative phosphorylation (ATP) production, mitochondrial dysfunction
    in sepsis and, 572–573
ARG1. See *Arginase 1 (ARG1).*
Arginase 1 (ARG1), depletion of, myeloid cells after, 495–496
Arginine
    deficiency of
        after PI, 492
        biologic function effects of, 492–495
    depletion of
        MDSC in correction of, 496–497
        myeloid cells after, 495–496
    dietary supplementation of, clinical studies of, 497–498
Arginine deficiency syndrome, 498
Aspiration, GRVs and, in critical illness, 485–486
ATP production. See *Altered oxidative phosphorylation (ATP) production.*

B

Biologic functions, arginine deficiency effects on, 492–495

C

Cellular metabolism/apoptosis, GLN in, 517
Cellular-organ protection, GLN in, 516–517
Clinical guidelines, described, 451
Critical illness
    energy expenditure during, variations in, 444
    fish oil in, **501–514**
    GLN in, **515–525.** See also *Glutamine (GLN), in critical illness.*
    GRVs in, **481–490.** See also *Gastric residual volumes (GRVs), in critical illness.*
    gut protection in, **549–565**
    omega-3 fatty acids in, **501–514.** See also *Omega-3 fatty acids.*
    PN in, outcome effects of, **467–480.** See also *Parenteral nutrition (PN), in critical illness,*
        outcome effects of.
Cytopathic hypoxia, microvascular dysfunction vs., mitochondrial dysfunction
    in sepsis and, 571

E

EBM. See *Evidence-based medicine (EBM).*
EGF. See *Epidermal growth factor (EGF).*
EN. See *Enteral nutrition (EN).*
Energy expenditure, during critical illness

Crit Care Clin 26 (2010) 577–582
doi:10.1016/S0749-0704(10)00051-5
0749-0704/10/$ – see front matter © 2010 Elsevier Inc. All rights reserved.
criticalcare.theclinics.com

Moving?

Make sure your subscription moves with you!

To notify us of your new address, find your **Clinics Account Number** (located on your mailing label above your name), and contact customer service at:

Email: journalscustomerservice-usa@elsevier.com

800-654-2452 (subscribers in the U.S. & Canada)
314-447-8871 (subscribers outside of the U.S. & Canada)

Fax number: 314-447-8029

Elsevier Health Sciences Division
Subscription Customer Service
3251 Riverport Lane
Maryland Heights, MO 63043

*To ensure uninterrupted delivery of your subscription, please notify us at least 4 weeks in advance of move.

Printed in the United States
By Bookmasters